SRI GARIB DASS ORIENTAL SERIES NO. 163

Gaṅgeśa on Yogarūḍhi

(Containing the original Text of the *Yogarūḍhivāda* of the *Śabdakhaṇḍa* of the *Tattvacintāmaṇi* with its English Translation and a detailed Introduction)

SUBAS CHANDRA DASH

SRI SATGURU PUBLICATIONS
A Division of
INDIAN BOOKS CENTRE
DELHI—INDIA

Published by :
SRI SATGURU PUBLICATIONS
A Division of
INDIAN BOOKS CENTRE
Indological & Oriental Publishers
40/5, Shakti Nagar
Delhi-110007
(INDIA)

First Edition : Delhi 1992

ISBN 81-7030-354-0

Printed in India :
Sainion Printary
Delhi-110053.

DEDICATED TO

THE FEET OF

MY REVERED GURU

Professor V.N. JHA

Foreword

It gives me great pleasure in writing a Foreword to this work of Dr. Subas Dash. Dr. Dash has received training in *Navya Nyāya* in the Centre of Advanced Study in Sanskrit, University of Poona. The present work has been prepared under my supervision. Dr. Dash has taken sufficient labour to work on the Concept of *Yogarūḍhi*. After thoroughly studying the section on *Yogarūḍhi* in the *Tatvacintāmaṇi* of Gaṅgeśopādhyāya and after presenting a readable translation of the text in English with notes wherever necessary in the second part, Dr. Dash has presented his detailed study, in part I, where he has given a brief history of the development of the Concept of *Yogarūḍhi* in Indian tradition. This is how the study has contributed to the furtherance of the study of the Concept of *Yogarūḍhi*.

The study provides the exact parameter for classification of words of a language in general and of Sanskrit in particular. The study reveals that there has been a long controversy over the acceptance of the category of *Yogarūḍhi śabda* and it discusses the logic for and against accepting such category. This study, I am sure, will be appreciated by Linguists as well, because it provides sufficient data to start meaningful interaction between scientific texts in Sanskrit and Philosophy of Language and similar material outcome in the Western thought. I am hopeful that the recent work will attract the attention of scholars in allied modern fields to take up studies of *Navya Nyāya* more seriously.

V.N. JHA
Director, Centre of Advanced
Study in Sanskrit,
University of Poona,
Pune—411007.

Foreword

It gives me great pleasure in writing a Foreword to this work of Dr. [illegible]. Dr. [illegible] has received training at [illegible] in the Centre of Advanced Study in Sanskrit, University of Poona. The present work has been prepared under my supervision. Dr. [illegible] has taken sufficient labour to work on the Concept of *Yogarūḍha*. After thoroughly studying the section on *Yogarūḍha* in the [illegible] of [illegible] and after presenting a readable translation of the text in English with notes wherever necessary in the second part, Dr. [illegible] has presented his critical study in part I wherein he has given a brief history of the development of the concept of *Yogarūḍha* in [illegible] tradition. This shows the study has contributed to the furtherance of the study of the Concept of *Yogarūḍha*.

The study provides the exact parameter for classification of words of a language in general and of Sanskrit in particular. The study reveals that there has been a long controversy over the acceptance of the category of *Yogarūḍha śabda* and it discusses the logic for and against accepting such category. This study, I am sure, will be appreciated by Linguists as well, because it provides sufficient data to start meaningful interaction between scientific texts in Sanskrit and Philosophy of Language and similar material outcome in the Western thought. I am hopeful that the present work will attract the attention of scholars in allied modern fields to take up studies of *Nyāya* [illegible] more seriously.

V. N. JHA
Director, Centre of Advanced
Study in Sanskrit,
University of Poona,
Pune—411007.

Preface

The present work is the revised version of my Ph.D. Thesis submitted to the University of Poona in 1990. The book is divided into two parts. In part—I, a detailed introduction is given where I have discussed various concepts of Nyāya which are related for the study of the concept of *Yogarūḍhi.* Śaśadhara, the Pre-Gaṅgeśa Navya-Naiyāyika has also discussed this problem of *Yogarūḍhi* in his text *Nyāyasiddhāntadīpa.* A reference is made to the arguments of Śaśadhara for comparison. It is proved that Gaṅgeśa of Śaśadhara those arguments of Śaśadhara in detail and after examining he gives his own view regarding the acceptance of *Yogarūḍhi.* In part—II, I have given a free English rendering of the *Yogarūḍhivāda* of the *śabdakhaṇḍa* of the *Tattvacintāmaṇi* of Gaṅgeśopādhyāya. The entire Sanskrit text has been divided into 172 passages from the standpoint of the logical presentation of the arguments.

I express my deep sense of respect and gratefulness to my *guru* Prof. V.N. Jha, Director, Centre of Advanced Study in Sanskrit, University of Poona who has guided me for preparing this thesis. It is all due to him that I could study the fundamentals of *Nyāya* which gave me a proper direction in this field.

I am obliged to Prof. S.D. Joshi, Ex-Director, CASS. University of Poona for giving me an opportunity to work in the Centre.

I have been benefited from the fatherly love and affection, inspirations and guidance of Paṇḍit T.S. Srinivas Shastri. I am very much grateful to him.

I express my thankfulness to Prof. Ashok Kelkar and Dr. Baliram Shukla for their constructive suggestions.

It is very difficult to put it in language my indebtedness to my parents, Father-in-law and family members whose love and affection and moral advice enabled me to come up to this stage. I cannot forget to keep on record my gratefulness to my wife Smt. Shantipriya Dash for the sacrifice rendered by her by relieving me of the domestic responsibilities and simultaneously helping me directly in my academic pursuits.

I am also very much thankful to my friends Dr. Kashinath Hota, Dr. Sasadhar Sahoo, Dr. Banamali Biswal, Mr. Suddhatattva Kar, Miss Kumuda Iyengar for their help during the preparation of this work.

I am sincerely thankful to the staff of the CASS Library, Jayakar Library, Bhandarkar Oriental Research Institute Library and Deccan College Library for their cordial help.

Finally, I also thank Indian Books Centre for taking up the publication of this work.

SUBAS CHANDRA DASH

Devasnāna Pūrnimā
June, 1992

Contents

Abbreviations

Kā. Sū. Vṛ.	—	*Kāvyālaṁkāra sūtra vṛttiḥ*
Kir.	—	*Kiraṇāvalī*
Tat. Ci. (Śabda)	—	*Tattvacintāmaṇi (Śabdakhaṇḍa)*
Tattvā. Sū.	—	*Tattvārtha Sūtra*
Tan. Var.	—	*Tāntravārttika*
Tar. Kau.	—	*Tarkakaumudī*
Tar. Dīp.	—	*Tarka Dīpikā*
Tar. Bhā.	—	*Tarka Bhāṣā*
Tar. Sam.	—	*Tarka Saṁgraha*
Nī. tat. bhā.	—	*Nītitattvāvirbhāva*
Nyā. Kan.	—	*Nyāya Kandalī*
Nyā. Ko.	—	*Nyāya Kośa*
Nyā. Dar.	—	*Nyāya Darśana*
Nyā. Pra.	—	*Nyāya Pradīpa*
Nyā. Bo.	—	*Nyāya Bodhinī*
Nyā. Bhā.	—	*Nyāya Bhāṣya*
Nyā. Bhū.	—	*Nyāya Bhūṣaṇa*
Nyā. Mañ.	—	*Nyāyamañjarī*
Nyā. Vār.	—	*Nyāya Vārttikam*
Nyā. Vār. Tāt Ṭīkā.	—	*Nyāya Vārttika Tātparya Ṭīkā*
Nyā. Si. Dī.	—	*Nyāyasiddhānta Dīpa*
Nyā. Bin. Ṭīkā	—	*Nyāya Bindu Ṭīkā*

Nyā. Mā. Vis.	—	*Nyāyamālā Vistara*
Nyā. Si. Mañ.	—	*Nyāyasiddhānta Mañjarī*
Nyā. Si. Mañ. Ṭī.	—	*Nyāyasiddhānta Mañjarī-Ṭīkā*
Nyā. Si. Muk.	—	*Nyāyasiddhānta Muktāvalī*
Nyā. Sū.	—	*Nyāya Sūtra*
Pra. Pañ	—	*Prakaraṇa Pañcikā*
Pras. Bhā.	—	*Praśastapāda Bhāṣya*
Bhā. Ci.	—	*Bhāṭṭa Cintāmaṇi*
Bhā. Kau.	—	*Bhāṭṭakaustubha*
Bau. Tar. Bhā.	—	*Bauddha Tarka Bhāṣā*
Bhā. Di	—	*Bhāṭṭa Dīpikā*
Bhā. Par.	—	*Bhāṣā Pariccheda*
Brah. Sū. Bhā.	—	*Brahma-Sūtra Bhāṣya*
Ma. Bhā.	—	*Mahābhāṣya*
Ma. Bhā. Pra.	—	*Mahābhāṣya Pradīpa*
Māme.	—	*Mānameyodaya*
Mīm. Sū.	—	*Mīmāṁsā Sūtra*
Rat. Dar.	—	*Ratna Darpaṇa*
Rasa.	—	*Rasagaṅgādhara*
Laghu. Mañ.	—	*Laghumañjuṣā*
La. Śa.	—	*Laghuśabdendu Śekhara*
Śakti.	—	*Śaktivāda*
Śab. Śa.	—	*Śabdaśaktiprakāśikā*
Śāb. Bhā.	—	*Śābara Bhāṣya*
Ślo. Vār.	—	*Ślokavārttika*
Sa. Kaṇ.	—	*Sarasvatīkaṇṭhābharaṇa*
Sām. Kār.	—	*Sāṁkhya Kārikā*
Sām. Tat. Kau.	—	*Sāṁkhya Tattva Kaumudī*

Śās. Dīp.	—	*Śāstra Dīpikā.*
Si. Ca.	—	*Siddhānta Candrodaya*
Sar. Dar. Saṁ.	—	*Sarva Darśana Saṁgraha*
Vāk.	—	*Vākyapadīya*
Veda Bhā. Bhā	—	*Veda Bhāskara Bhāṣya*
Vai. Bhū.	—	*Vaiyākaraṇa Bhūsaṇasāra*
Vai. Sū. Upas	—	*Vaiśeṣika Sūtropaṣkāra*
Vai. Sū.	—	*Vaiśeṣika Sūtra*
Vyut.	—	*Vyutpattivāda*
JOIB.	—	*Journal of the Oriental Institute, Baroda*

Part I

Introduction

0.0. PLAN OF WORK

Among four *pramāṇas* the *Śabdapramāṇa* generates verbal understanding. The Naiyāyikas argue in favour of a particular process of verbal understanding. They hold that a sentence possessed of *ākāṅkṣā*, *yogyatā* and *sannidhi* along with *tātparya* generates verbal understanding. But these factors are not enough for that purpose. These factors can work provided the relation between a word and its meaning is known. This relation is called *vṛtti.* This problem is not only the problem of the Naiyāyikas, but also of the Mīmāṁsakas, Grammarians and those who deal with the process of verbal understanding. So the relation between a word and its meaning plays an important role in Indian philosophy. According to the Naiyāyikas—*vṛtti* is of two types namely—*śakti* and *lakṣaṇā*. *Śakti* is the primary relation and *lakṣaṇā* is the secondary relation. The primary relation again is divided into four types namely—(i) *yoga* (ii) *rūḍhi* (iii) *yogarūḍhi* and (iv) *yaugikarūḍhi.* Accordingly the words are also divided into four types namely—

(i) *yaugika* (ii) *rūḍha* (iii) *yogarūḍha* and (iv) *yaugikarūḍha*.

In this thesis an attempt is made to study the philosophy and the arguments advanced for or against *yogarūḍhi*, as a third type of the primary relation. For this purpose, the textual portion of the *Yogarūḍhivāda* from the *Śabdakhaṇḍa* of Gaṅgeśa's *Tattvacintāmaṇi* is taken up. I have translated the whole text in English with explanatory notes wherever necessary. I have divided the extent of my thesis into two parts. In the first part, a long introduction dealing with various concepts regarding *śabdapramāṇa* is discussed. I am going to discuss the various types of words and its classification and the relationship between a word and its meaning. Here I have also devoted a separate chapter to the history and development of the concept of *yogarūḍhi* in Indian Philosophy.

The arguments in favour of *yogarūḍhi* in the system other than the Nyāya-Vaiśeṣika is also taken into consideration. The pre-Gaṅgeśa author, Śaśadhara who has also dealt with the problem in a great detail, has been consulted for the present thesis. An attempt has also been made to compare the similar concepts in modern linguistics. And after that follow my observations. The second part of the thesis includes the text of *Yogarūḍhivāda* along with the English translation and explanatory notes.

0.1. GENERAL CONCEPT OF PRAMĀṆA

In Indian philosophy the concept of *pramāṇa* plays an important role in the field of epistemological analysis. The word *pramāṇa* is a bit ambiguous.

(*i*) When its derivative structure has an instrumental form e.g. *pramīyate jñāyate anena*, it signifies the means of valid cognition and the word *pramāṇa* is always used in this normal sense.

(*ii*) On the otherhand, when its derivative structure has a *bhāva* form, it signifies the knowledge itself *pramiṇoti iti pramāṇam*.

So various systems of Indian philosophy interprets the word *pramāṇa* as a valid cognition and also a means or an instrument of valid cognition. Some systems identify the two concepts of *pramā* and *pramāṇa* as well. But the *Naiyāyīkas* strictly maintain and use the word *pramā* as valid cognition and *pramāṇa* as the means of valid cognition. While discussing the concept *pramāṇa* as understood by various systems the identity and the difference between the two are well maintained.

The *pramāṇas* are the instruments of valid cognitions. One *pramāṇa* corresponds to one cognition e.g. *pratyakṣa pramāṇa* is the instrument for producing the resultant perceptual cognition.

(1) *Cārvāka School*

The Cārvākas recognise one source of knowledge i.e. *pratyakṣa* 'Perception'. They do not rely upon any other knowledges like inferential cognition etc. Only the perceptual cognition of an object is real for them. The other things which cannot be perceived through sense organs, are unreal according to them. So naturally, the chances of other *pramāṇas* don't stand at all. That is why they accept one type of cognition—i.e. perception and hence there is one instrument or means of valid knowledge i.e. *pratyakṣa.*

(2) *Vaiśeṣika School*

The Vaiśeṣikas advocate only two *pramāṇas* namely :

(i) Perception (*pratyakṣa*)	and	(ii) Inference (*anumāna*)

They define *pramāṇa* as the operative cause *karaṇa* or instrument of both the memory and experience.[1] Kaṇāda mentions that the general definition of *pramāṇa* should be based on the principle that the cause of cognition (*vidyā*) should be free from defects.[2] The Veda Bhāṣkara Bhāṣya records that when the sense-organs are without faults, the (*saṁskāras*) impressions become also faultless. And only when the impressions are present, the real knowledge of objects occurs. That *vidyā* (knowledge) is only generated or grasped by *pramāṇa* which is free from defects.[3]

Praśastapāda includes perception, inference and *ārṣa* under *vidyā*, and illusion under *avidyā*. In his *bhāṣya* we don't find any clear-cut definition of *pramāṇa.*

Śrīdhara refers to another factor '*adhyavasāya*' meaning that *vidyā* is a definite cognition.[4]

Śaṁkara Mishra, in his *Upaskāra* on the *Vai. sū.*, however mentions that, a *pramāṇa* is that which produces true knowledge.[5]

(3) *Buddhist School*

According to the Buddhist philosophy, a *pramāṇa* is not

different from the resultant knowledge *pramā*. Dharmakirti in the beginning of his text *Nyāyabindu* mentions the word *samyag-jñāna* which stands for *pramāṇa*. In *Tīkā*, Dharmottara mentions that *pramāṇa* is an uncontradicted experience.[6]

In *Buddha Tarkabhāṣā*, Mokṣākara Gupta holds the same view. He says that the knowledge is called as *pramāṇa* in which the object is not known earlier.[7] The term is explained as that cognition which leads to the obtainment of the same object shown by that cognition.[8] As it is further clarified that, *pramāṇa* is that in which the object is not known.[9] So the meaning of the term *avisaṁvādaka* is that cognition which leads to inconsistant behaviour.

Some philosophers say that the sense organs are insensient and therefore it cannot generate knowledge. It is only the earlier knowledge which gives birth to a subsequent knowledge and the chain continues. This school clearly holds the view that consciousness *vijñāna* itself is *pramāṇa*.[10]

The Buddhists argue that the object is nothing but the objectification of the individual consciousness. The yellow, red and blue coloured objects are nothing but the consciousness of the yellow, red and blue colours. It is only the red consciousness or the yellow consciousness which takes an objective form.

But the Naiyāyika's don't accept the arguments given by the Idealists with regard to the concept of *pramāṇa* and proves that *pramāṇa* is the instrument and *pramā* is the resultant knowledge.[11] However, the Buddhists accept two *pramāṇas* (i) perception and (ii) Inference.

The realistic schools of Buddhist philosophy namely—the *Sautrāntika* and the *Vaibhāṣika* define *pramāṇa* as the knowledge with a form of an object which is identical with the knowledge and the object of it.[12] For example—the knowledge of red colour is not only through the action of eyes etc., but it is the red content of the object that determines our knowledge of a red colour. The content of the object of a knowledge gives rise to the knowledge of the same content, and thereby reveals the object itself as having that content. This is called the *arthākāra* or *sākāra* which is the *pramāṇa.* Here the content of the object is both the means and the result of the knowledge. That is to say—a cognition becomes valid when it has the same content as the object cognised by it. In other words, the content of an object *arthākāra* is *pramāṇa* in so far as it establishes an identity between the object and our knowledge of it. *Ākāra* and *ākārin* are different aspects of the same entity.

(4) *Nyāya School*

What is pramāṇa ?

A *pramāṇa* is defined as an instrument by which something is rightly known. In other words a *pramāṇa* is an instrument of *pramā.*[13] With reference to such derivative structure of *pramāṇa*, it naturally refers to instrumentality. That is why Vātsyāyana has rightly defined in another way that—the *pramāṇas* refer to the instrumental cause of valid knowledge.[14]

This suggests that from a group of causes any cause cannot be treated as *pramāṇa.* Only an instrumental cause can be a *pramāṇa.* But how to know this *kāraṇa* ? The logicians provide a rule that is only treated as a cause which invariably and immediately precedes the effect.[15] As there are many causes only one among them which is of a specific nature and uncommon must be treated as *kāraṇa* and that is *kāraṇa* and also that is treated as *pramāṇa.* *Pāṇini* defines *kāraṇā* as *sādhakatamam*, i.e. an instrument which is the most excellent (effective) factor among a group of factors to produce the result.

To this, we can say that it is the extra-ordinary cause (factor) of an effect which is different from the other ordinary factors. In fact, only the instrumental cause (*kāraṇa*) can be considered to be the most efficient one. But how to know a particular factor to be the most efficient among a group of factors ?

The Naiyāyikas therefore suggest that, no doubt there are many factors which come together to produce an effect. But some are related closely to the effect than others. To be precise, some causes are most important, active for producing the effect, while others simply play their role individually, directly or indirectly.

But an extra-ordinary cause is directly connected to the effect. For this the logicians provide two different definitions of *kāraṇa* as follows :

(I) *Ist definition*

vyāpāravadasādhāraṇam kāraṇam karaṇam.

According to this definition a cause which is extra-ordinary (un-common) and which possesses *vyāpāra* is known as *karaṇa.* For example :

X produces Y and Y produces Z

$X \rightarrow Y \rightarrow Z$

Here X produces Y which also produces Z. According to the definition—*tadjjanyatve sati tradjjanyajanakatvam vyāpāratvam.* Y is called as *vyāpāra* which produces Z (*phala*). Naturally a *vyāpāra* requires two factors :

(i) It should be produced by something and

(ii) It also produces something.

And *vyāpāravat* is that which possesses *vyāpāra* i.e. 'X' here, which is *asādhāraṇa kāraṇa* for producing the effect 'Z'. This *vyāpāravat* immediately brings result is the opinion of the Old Nyāya School.

(II) *IInd definition*

phalāyogavyavacchinnam kāraṇam karaṇam

This second definition states that a cause which is not dissociated from the effect is known as *karaṇa*. And that *karaṇa* is called *pramāṇa*. Here in the above example X produces Y and Y produces Z, Y is the cause. By the help of two negative expressions Y becomes the *karaṇa*. So Y produces Z directly and hence Y is treated as *pramāṇa* is the explanation given by the neo-logicians.

There may be a difference of opinion between the Old and the New school of Naiyāyikas. But it is a fact that all the Naiyāyīkas agree that a *pramāṇa* is *karaṇa* which is the instrumental and the most efficient cause of valid knowledge.

In Nyāya-Vaiśeṣika system there are four factors which are necessary for the production of a valid knowledge. They are enumerated by Vātsyāyana in his *Nyāya Bhāṣya* (*Nyā. Bhā*) as follows.[16]

There is a knower—*pramātṛ* one who has a volition, who is desirous of getting something and desirous of giving up something. There is a knowable—*prameya* i.e. an object to be known, the knower gets the knowledge of that object i.e. *pramiti* and there is an instrument through which it is known i.e. *pramāṇa.*

In Nyāya system there are four *pramāṇas* namely :

(1) *Pratyakṣa pramāṇa* (Perceptual Instrument)

(2) *Anumāna pramāṇa* (Inferential Instrument)

(3) *Upamāna pramāṇa* (Analogical Instrument)

(4) *Śabda pramāṇa* (Verbal Instrument)

Corresponding to these above four *pramāṇas*, the four types of knowledges are generated. They are as follows :

(1) *Pratyakṣa* (Perception or Perceptual Knowledge)

(2) *Anumiti* (Inference or Inferential Knowledge)

(3) *Upamiti* (Analogy or Analogical Knowledge)

(4) *Śābdabodha* (Verbal Testimony or Verbal Knowledge)

Gautama, the founder of Nyāya School does not give any definition of *pramāṇa*. But the very idea of *pramāṇa* is introduced in his *Nyāya-Sūtra* (*Nyā. Sū.*). In the definition of *upamāna* the reference of the concept of *pramāṇa* is very well-judged.[17] That means a *pramāṇa* is that which produces the knowledge of *sādhya*. Such a knowledge may be either a perceptual knowledge or an inferential knowledge or an analogical or verbal knowledge.

Vātsyāyana refers to the notion of *pramāṇa* as the instrument of knowledge.[18] He further clarifies by supplying *sa (pramātā) yena artham pramiṇoti tat pramāṇam.* He also mentions that *pramāṇa* always apprehends things as they are.[19] In another context while discussing the nature of *pramāṇa* he directly refers that *pramāṇas* are the sources of cognition.[20]

From the time of Uddyotakara onwards we find that the Naiyāyikas have tried to give a formal definition of *pramāṇa*. He defines it as the cause of knowledge or the source of knowledge.[21]

Then comes Vācaspati Mishra. He replaces the word *upalabdhi* by *pramā* and the definition given by him is—*pramā sādhanam hi pramāṇam.*[22]

Udayana and other Naiyāyikas except Jayanta Bhaṭṭa belonging to both old and new schools have followed this improved definition of *pramāṇa* suggested by Vācaspati Mishra.

It is a fact that those who say that *pramāsādhanam pramāṇam* think of a particular *kāraka* as *pramāṇa*. Therefore eyes or its contact with the object can be the *pramāṇa* for perceptual knowledge, a probans will be the *pramāṇa* for inferential knowledge, the knowledge of similarity for the analogical knowledge, and the knowledge of words for the verbal knowledge.

Whatever may be the various ways of defining *pramāṇa* stated earlier, Jayanta, a poet-Naiyāyika, puts forward an altogether different concept of *pramāṇa*.[23] His theory says that no single *kāraka* or instrument produces result. But it is a collection of factors or *kārakas* which produce result. Therefore, this collection of factors or *sāmagrī* is *pramāṇa*. He defines it in the following manner : *avyabhicāriṇīmasandigdhāmarthopalabdhim vidadhatī bodhābodhasvabhāva sāmagrī pramāṇam.*[24] That means a collection of factors which is both of the nature of knowledge and of the nature of non-knowledge and which generates the knowledge of an object which must be correct and undoubtful is called *pramāṇa*.

Here in this definition *sāmagrī* is *kāraṇa* and that *karaṇa* is *pramāṇa*. From this definition we can say that, *pramāṇa* denotes a group of conditions which can be divided into two categories :

(i) some are partly physical and

(ii) some are partly psychical in nature.

For example : The perceptual knowledge of a pot requires the physical contact between the eyes and the pot (*indrīyārtha sannikarśa*) and so also by the internal physical process (operations) of the contact of the *Ātman* with the mind (*ātmā manasā saṁyujyate*).

(5) *Mimāṁsā School*

The . .ābhākara school of Pūrva-mīmāṁsā accepts five *pramāṇas* namely—(1) *pratyakṣa* (2) *anumāna* (3) *upamāna* (4) *śabda* and (5) *arthāpatti* (implication).

But the Bhāṭṭa school accepts one more in addition to the above five—that is *abhāva* 'absence.'

According to Prābhākaras cognition has been divided into two categories—as (1) valid and (2) invalid. The valid cognitions are those which directly connected with the objects and invalid cognitions are those which are related with objects indirectly. *Anubhūti* 'experience' comes under valid cognition and *smṛti* 'remembrance' comes under invalid cognition.

The Prābhākaras understand *pramāṇa* in the sense of valid cognition. They define this valid cognition as—*pramāṇa* is experience (*anubhūti*) which is different from remembrance which is not valid which requires an earlier cognition to occur, being it as a cognition produced only by the impressions left by a previous cognition.[25] They identify *pramāṇa* with *pramā*. According to them all cognitions are valid and their invalidity is due to their dis-agreement with the real nature of their subjects.

They say that *pramāṇa* is that which gives us new knowledge i.e. a valid knowledge of objects of which we have had no knowledge in the past. *Pramāṇa* is the means to have the knowledge of something of that object which are not known. If it is already known, then there is no necessity of knowing it again through a process. The method is therefore related to the process of knowing what has not been previously known. That is why memory '*smṛti* has been excluded from the area of *pramā* because it is not a new experience rather a recollection of some old experience.[26]

According to Kumārila Bhaṭṭa *pramāṇa* is a definite and assured cognition of objects which does not require confirmation by other cognitions and at the same time it is inferred on the basis of *dṛṣṭatā* produced in an object. He mentions that a cognition as means of valid cognition (*pramāṇa*), because it comes under experience. He regards cognizedness (*jñātatā*) produced by a cognitive act as its result. Kumārila holds that a knowledge, an act of the self, is *pramāṇa* which is inferred from its result or cognizedness.

(6) *Vedānta School*

Śankarācārya puts forth almost some views regarding the concept of *pramāṇa*.[27] That means the knowledge is generated by the help of *pramāṇa* and *pramāṇa* is that which presents the content as it is.

The Vedānta school admits six *pramāṇas* namely: (1) perception (2) Inference (3) Analogy (4) Verbal Testimony (5) *Arthāpatti* and (6) *abhāva* (Absence).

(7) *Sāṁkhya School*

The Sāṁkhya school admits three *pramāṇas* namely: (1) Perception (2) Inference and (3) Verbal Testimony.

The *Sāṁkhyakārikā* mentions there are three *pramāṇas*.[28] Īśvarakṛṣṇa does not define *pramāṇa* explicitly, but he uses the term *pramāṇa*. Where as Vācaspati Mishra thinks that Īśvarakṛṣṇa does not define *pramāṇa* because of its derivative nature. Through derivation he means that 'through which knowledge arises' and hence *pramāṇa* is regarded as a source of valid knowledge. He mentions that the result is the valid knowledge and the means is *pramāṇa*.[29]

(8) *Yoga School*

The Yoga system accepts three types of *pramāṇas* namely: (1) perception (2) Inference and (3) Verbal Testimony like Sāṁkhya school.[30] Patañjali in his *Yoga Sūtra* holds the view that *pramāṇa* is one of the functions of *citta*.[31]

This definition is very old and does not seem to be influenced by the epistemology of Nyāya-Vaiśeṣika. Patañjali however shows superiority of yogic practices and consequently yogic perception acquired through them over ordinary means of knowledge. He says that *Buddhi* through the discipline of Yoga gets truth—bearing knowledge (*ṛtambharā*) having no reference to wrong or perverted knowledge.[32]

This knowledge comprehends particularly *viśeṣa* residing in *puruṣa* or in subtle elements which is not known through any of the worldly means of knowledge.[33]

(9) *Jaina School*

A different kind of approach towards the definition of *pramāṇa* is given by the Jaina philosophers. In his work *Nyāyāvatāra*, Siddhasena Divākara clearly mentions that a *pramāṇa* is defined as knowledge which illumines itself and other objects (*sva-para*) and is without any obstruction.[34] Here also the knowledge i.e. the result or effect of *pramāṇa* is treated as *pramāṇa* itself.

The Jaina School records five kinds of knowledges[35] namely:

(1) Ordinary knowledge obtained by sense-perception (*mati*)

(2) Scriptural knowledge (*śṛuti*)

(3) Knowledge of things even at a distance of time and space (*avadhi*)

(4) Knowledge of thoughts of others (*manaḥ-paryāya*) and

(5) Omniscience (*Kevala*)

The first two are called indirect (*parokṣa*), because they are obtained with the external help of the sense organs on scripture. And the last three are direct (*pratyakṣa*), because they are obtained directly by the soul without any external help of the sense-organs nor by mind or scripture. These two direct and indirect knowledges are recognised as two sets of *pramāṇas*.[36]

Now a question arises what determines the number of the sources or means of *pramāṇas*. Obviously, this will be the answer : the nature of the object of knowledge determines the number of the source of knowledge. A particular object is revealed by a specific source of knowledge. Hence the number of the source of knowledge depends on the nature of the object. If there is one kind of knowledge which is perceivable then it is to be known by perception only. As there are various objects of knowledges there follows also number of sources of knowledge by which those objects are grasped.

It is the nature of knowledge that determines the nature of the process through which a particular knowledge comes into existence and the difference in the process amounts to the difference in the number of *pramāṇas*, as many valid processes so many *pramāṇas*.

Notes

1. *smṛtyanubhavasādhāraṇam pramākaraṇam pramāṇam, Tar Kau*, p. 15.
2. *aduṣṭam vidyā. Vai. Sū. with Veda Bhā. Bhā.* 9.2.12. p. 237.
3. *nirdoṣendriyeṣu nirdoṣā bhavanti saṁskārāḥ. tataśca sadbhūtārthajñānam jāyate. sā vidyā pramāṇāya bhavati. Veda Bhā. Bhā*, p. 238.

4. *niḥsandigdhābādhītādhyavasāyātmikā pratītirvidyā. Nyā. Kan*, p. 414.
5. *aduṣṭamaduṣṭendriyajanyam yatra yadasti tatra tadanubhavo vā, sāmānādhikaraṇa prakārānubhavo vā, viśeṣyāvṛtyaprakārakānubhavo vā, vidyetyarthaḥ, Vai. Sū. Upas.* on 9.2.12, p. 518.
6. *avisaṁvādakam jñānam samyagjñānam, Nyā. Bin. Ṭīkā*, p. 1ɔ.
7. *pramāṇam samyagjñānamapūrvagocaram, pramīyate, rtho, neneti pramāṇam, tadeva samyagjñānam, Bau. Tar. Bhā.* p. 1.
8. *loke ca pūrvamupadarśitamartham, prāpayat saṁvādakamuchyate, Nyā. Bin. Ṭīkā*, p. 10.
9. *ataeva ca anadhigata viṣayam pramāṇam.* Ibid., p. 11.
10. *vijñānasyaivānākārasyātmānātmaprakāśanasāmarthyamityapare. Nyā. Vār. Tāt. Ṭīkā*, p. 15.
11. *Pramāṇa* portion, Jayanta's. *Mañ.* Ist. Āhnika.
12. *viṣayasārūpyam sākārasya vijñānasyetyanye. Nyā. Vār. Tāt. Ṭīkā*, p. 15.
13. *pramīyateneneti karaṇārthābhidhāno hi pramāna śabdaḥ Nyā. Bhā.* 1.1.3, p. 91.
14. *Upalabdhisādhnāni pramāṇāni*, Ibid.
15. *Kāryaniyatapūrvavartitvam kāraṇatvam.*
16. *tatra yasyepsājihāsāprayuktasya pravṛttiḥ sa pramātā, sa yenārtham pramiṇoti tatpramāṇam, yo'rthaḥ pramīyate tat prameyam, yad arthavijñānam sā pramītiḥ, catasṛṣu caivam vidhāsvartha tattvam parisamāpyate. Nyā. Dar.* 1.1.1., p. 24.
17. *prasiddhasādharmyāt sādhyasādhanamupamānam. Nyā. Sū.*, 1.1.6.
18. *pramāṇataḥ arthapratipattau pravṛttisāmarthyāt arthavat pramāṇam. Nyā. Bhā.* on 1.1.1.
19. *yathābhānaviṣayakam hi pramāṇamiti, Nyā. Bhā.* 3.1.51.
20. *upalabdhisādhanāni pramāṇāni. Nyā Bhā.* 1.1.3.
21. *upalabdhi hetuḥ pramāṇam, upalabdhihetutvam pramāṇatvam. Nyā. Vār.*, p. 15.
22. *Nyā. Tāt. Ṭīkā*, p. 16.

23. Cf. 'Jayanta's concept of *Pramāṇa* by Prof. V.N. *Jha. Studies in Language, Logic and Epistemology*, p. 26.
24. *Nyā. Mañ.* Vol. I. p. 31.
25. "*pramāṇamanubhūtiḥ*" *na ca smṛteḥ prāmāṇyāpattiriti darśayati*/ "*sā smṛteranyā na sā smṛtiḥ*".// *Pra. Pañ.* p. 124.
26. *yathārthamagṛhītagrāhijñānam pramāṇamiti. Sās. Dīp*, p. 75.
27. *jñānantu pramāṇajanyam pramāṇañca yathābhūta vastu viṣayakam. Brah. Sū. Bhā.* 1.1.4. p. 129.
28. *dṛṣṭamanumānamāptavacanam ca sarvapramāṇabiddhatvāt/ trividham pramāṇamiṣṭam prameyasiddhiḥ pramāṇāddhi*// *Sām. Kār.* 4.
29. *phalam pramā, tatsādhanam pramāṇamiti*/ *Sām. Tat. kau.* on *kārikā* 4.
30. *pratyakṣānumānāgamāḥ pramāṇāni. Yoga Sūtra*, 1.7.
31. *pramāṇa viparyayavikalpanidrā smṛtayaḥ*, Ibid. 1.6.
32. *ṛtambharā tatra prajñā*, Ibid. 1.48.
33. *Yoga Bhāṣya*, 1.49.
34. *pramāṇam svaparābhāsi jñānam bādhavivarjitam*/ *Nyāyāvatāra*, verse 1, p. 10.
35. *matisrutā'vadhimanaḥparyāyakevalāni jñānam. Tattvā. Sū.* 1.9.
36. Ibid. 1.10—11.

0.2. THE CONCEPT OF ŚABDAPRAMĀṆA

The Vaiśeṣikas do not accept *Śabda* as a separate *pramāṇa*, but include it under Inference. Kaṇāda however, did not make any reference to *śabdapramāṇa* in his *Vaiśeṣika sūtra*. As *śabda* gives the knowledge of something not perceivable by the sense organs, just like *anumāna*, *śabda* follows the same process as in the case of inference and hence it is included under inference.[1] At the time of Praśastapāda this statement is made clear. But it is much more clear from the *Upaskāra* of Śankara Mishra. He mentions that—

etena śābdam vyākhyātam. śābdam śabdakaraṇakam jñānamidam iti yannaiyāyikānāmbhimatam tadapyetena laiṅgikatvena laiṅgaprabhavatvena vyākhyātam. yathā vyāpti pakṣadharmatāpratisaṁdhānāpekṣam laiṅgikam tathā śābdamapi.

But we see that from the time of Praśastapāda onwards the discussion on *śabda* and the word meaning relationship[2] is widely analysed and they accept *samaya* as the relation. The long discussion on *avinābhāva sambandha* (*Vyāpti*) as the relation between word and its meaning is the view of the opponents. But from this we can say that, they were influenced to some extent by the Nyāya theory of *śabda*, eventhough they did not accept *śabda* as a separate type of *Pramāṇa*.

But the *śabdapramāṇa* is one among the four *pramāṇas* in Nyāya philosophy. Among four *pramāṇas*, the *śabdapramāṇa* generates verbal understanding. This verbal understanding occurs in the listener from a sentence when uttered by some one. It is also a fact that when the speaker utters a sentence the listener understands the meaning. That is why *śabda* is defined by Gautama[3] as *āptopadeśaḥ* i.e. as a statement of a trustworthy person. Annambhaṭṭa practically repeats the same as *āptavākyam śabdaḥ.*[4] Then naturally, question arises who is called on *āpta*? According to the Nyāya system an *āpta* is described as a preson who has knowledge of the reality and who speaks the truth.[5] He need not necessarily be an expert but he should be a speaker of truth or facts which give correct information about something when asked and not a cheat (*Vipralambhaka*). As *āpta* is regarded as a trust-worthy person who, never lies. The listener listens to him carefully with much belief. Vātsyāyana refers to the qualities or qualification of an *āpta*. These are :

(i) possession of relevant knowledge
(ii) integrity of motivation and
(iii) ability for adequate communication.[6]

"That person is called *āpta* 'reliable', who possesses the direct and right knowledge of things, who is moved by a desire to make known to others the things as he knows it, and who is fully capable of speaking of it." Let us analyse the above conditions further. The first condition does not inform that a person is an expert because the knowledge involved might be just an ordinary knowledge and not specialised or expert knowledge. In the second case, a man of integrity need not be an expert. Similar is the case with regard to the ability to communicate adequately, what is communicated need not be specialised or expert knowledge. Seeing an object with one's own eyes is called its *āpti*. The *āpta* is socalled because he acts with that i.e. with the *āpti* or direct apprehension of an object. The same definition holds good of all *āptas* whether *ṛṣis*, *āryas* or *mlecchas*.[7] That is why not all *śabdas* are capable of being proved to be true but only those *śabdas* which are voluntarily uttered by persons who have directly apprehended the objects referred to by the *śabdas*.

If we look to the definition given by Annambhaṭṭa, there is no suggestion of expert knowledge as the characteristic feature of an *āpta*. The truth mentioned or referred by *śabda* is just simple truth or matter of facts. Therefore, *āpta* has to be understood only as a reliable or trustworthy person and should not be treated as an expert.

Another point is to be noted here that, the Naiyāyīkas do not restrict the term *āpta* only to ordinary speakers but include God also as an *āpta*. There are two kinds of *śabda* namely— (i) *laukika* 'mundane' and (ii) *vaidika* or *alaukika* 'scriptural.'[8] And both of them are treated as *āptavacanas*. They say that the scriptural *śabda* is what is uttered by *Īśvara* while mundane *śabda* is uttered by a trustworthy person.

The *śabdapramāṇa* produces the *śābdabodha* (verbal understanding). For the verbal understanding *śabda* is not merely a cause but there are other factors which cause the remembrance of meaning of the sentence. The factors include *pada*, *padārtha*, *sambandha*, *vākyārtha* and also the intention of the speaker *tātparya* is equally, important. So also the concepts like (*yogyatā*) compatibility, (*ākāṅkṣā*) expectancy and (*sannidhi*) proximity are the indispensable elements of a sentence. These factors will be analysed separately in the forthcoming chapters to a great detail.

Notes

1. *tadvacanādāmnāyasya Prāmāṇyam*. Vai. Sū. 1.1.3.
2. (i) *yathā prasiddhasamayasyāsandigdhaliṅgadarśana prasiddhyanusmaraṇābhyāmatīndrīye'rthe bhavatyanumānameva śabdādibhyo'piti.*

   Pras. Bhā with *Nyā. Kan.* p. 512.

   (*ii*) *kīdṛśam tasya sambandhasya jñānam, asya śabdasyayamartho vācya ityevambhūta iti cet*. Ibid. p. 518.

   (iii) *samayaḥ sambandhamātram avyabhicāra iti yāvat*. *Kir*. p. 206.

   (iv) *samayaḥ īśvarasaṁketaḥ, Vai. Sū. Upas*. p. 430.

3. *Nyā. Sū.* 1.1.7.
4. *Tar Saṁ* p. 50.
5. *āptastu yathārthavaktā.* Ibid.
6. *āptaḥ khalu sākṣātkṛtadharmāyathādṛṣṭasyārthasya cikhyāpayiṣayā prayukta upadeṣṭā. Nyā. Bhā.* 1.1.7.
7. *sākṣātkaraṇamarthasyā'ptiḥ tayā pravartata ityāptaḥ ṛṣyāryamlecchānām samānam lakṣaṇam.* Ibid, p. 174.
8. *vākyam dvividham laukikam vaidikam ca. vaidikamīśvaroktatvātsarvameva pramāṇam, laukikamtvāptoktam pramāṇam. Tar. Saṁ* p. 53.

0.3. PROCESS OF VERBAL UNDERSTANDING

According to the Naiyāyikas the verbal understanding has a process. When a speaker utters a sentence the listener understands it and gets the meaning of that uttered sentence. They hold that a sentence possessed of *ākāṅkṣa*, *yogyatā* and *sannidhi* generates the verbal understanding.[1] These three factors are not enough for causing the verbal understanding. But over and above these factors there is a relation between the word and its meaning which plays an important role in the process of verbal understanding.

Now let us discuss in detail the above factors. Expectancy (*ākāṅkṣā*)[2] is defined as a particular sequence of words without which the *padas* are not capable of generating the verbal understanding. Viśvanātha Nyāyapañcānana elaborates on that point and says the samething in a different manner. When the *padas* are not arranged properly then there won't arise any understanding. Without a verb, there won't be any *kāraka* as such.[3] Suppose there is a word *pustakam*, if *pustaka* and the accusative suffix—*am* are written separately or uttered as—*am pustaka* then no one will be able to understand anything out of it. Hence there is a necessity of a sequence of these words for proper understanding and the factor of sequence or proper order (ānupūrvī) is called *ākāṅkṣā*.

Compatibility (*yogyatā*) is another factor without which verbal understanding does not arise. *Yogyatā* is defined as the feasibility of relation of one word meaning with another.[4] For instance, in the sentence *bahninā siñcati* (He) sprinkles with fire, there is no feasibility of the relation of the meaning of the word *bahni* with sprinkling with water. As a matter of fact, we experience that *jalena siñcati* '(He) sprinkles with water', there is feasibility of the relation of the meaning of the word *jala* with the meaning of the instrumental suffix namely *karaṇatva*, because sprinkling a plant with water is quite feasible.

Proximity (*sannidhi*) is defined as uttering the words in a sentence without any time gap.[5] If somebody utters the word *Devadattaḥ* today and the word *taṇḍulam* tomorrow and the word *pacati* the next day, then no one will have the verbal understanding that 'Devadatta cooks rice'. So the words of a sentence should be uttered or supplied at a regular interval of time. This factor is called *sannidhi* 'the proximity of words'.

Hence, if one knows these three factors of a sentence, where there are collection of words, then only he will have the verbal understanding on hearing or reading that sentence. Otherwise it is an impossible situation for the person to get verbal understanding. Hence, *śabda-pramāṇa* operates in such case but also one should be aware of the relationship between the words and their meanings as well. If this relation is not known the listener won't be able to get the verbal understanding. This relation is called *vṛtti*[6] which can be either *śakti* 'desire' or *lakṣaṇā* 'the relation with the primary meaning'. Let us call *śakti* as a primary relation or the expressive power of a word and *lakṣaṇā* as the secondary relation. It should be noted that the Nyāya-vaiśeṣika system does not need any other relation (*vṛtti*) in order to explain verbal understanding.

Now let us come to the proper process of the verbal under standing. A listener listens to a sentence or a reader reads a sentence. Since he knows the language he is also aware of the constituents (words) of that sentence and also the relation of the parts with their respective meanings. And after knowing the constituents he remembers their respective meanings. Here the *padajñāna* is the cause of *padārthasmaraṇa* and through the relation *śakti, śābdabodha* is generated.[7] While deciding the word meanings the listener decides the intention of the speaker and fixes the intended meanings of those constituents. And finally those remembered meanings form one integrated structure of the qualifier and qualificand type. The knowledge of this is what is called the verbal understanding.[8]

To put it differently—the knowledge of the words is the instrument (*karaṇa*), the knowledge of the *padārthas* is the *vyāpāra* or *dvāra* and *śābdabodha* is the verbal understanding which is the final result which is generated by the help of *śakti* or *lakṣaṇā*.

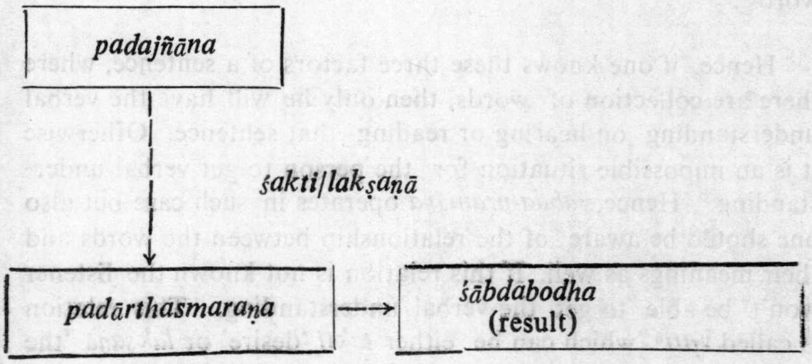

Suppose to take an example—in the sentence—*Rāmaḥ grāmam gacchati*. Here, the verbal understanding arises through a process which has been presented diagramatically. The first group of words generate the remembrance of meanings and then the respective meanings are related each other and finally the whole meaning of the sentence occurs as—'Rama goes to the village'.

This is the Naiyāyikas process of verbal understanding.

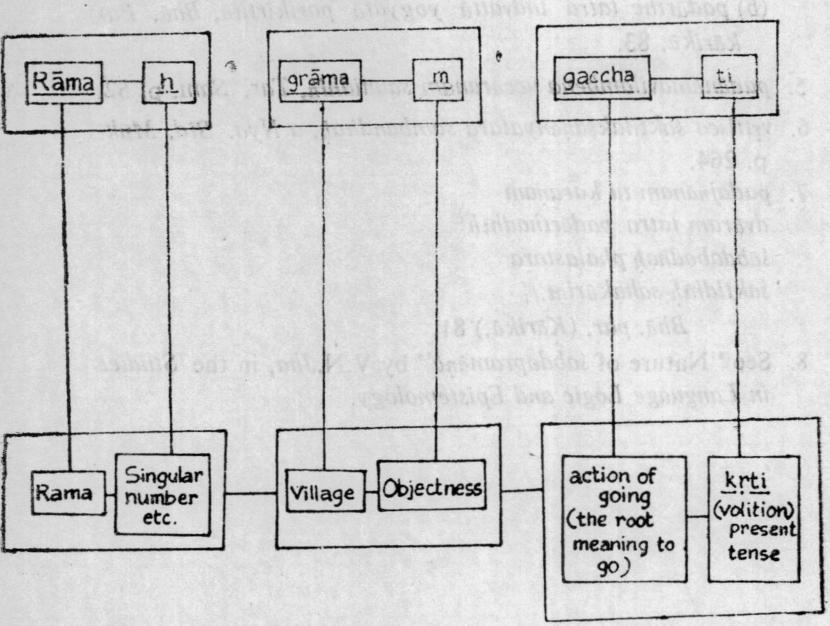

Notes

1. *ākāṅkṣā yogyatā sannidhiśca vākyārthajñānahetuḥ* Tar. Saṁ. p. 52.
2. (*a*) *Padasya padāntaravyatirekaprayuktānvayānanubhāvakatvamākāṅkṣā*—Ibid.
   (b) *yatpadena vinā yasyānanubhāvaktā bhavet ākāṅkṣā*. *Bhā. Par. Kārikā*. 84. p. 312.
3. *yena padena vinā yatpadasyānvayānanubhāvakatvam, tena padena saha tasyā "kāṅkṣetyarthaḥ, kriyāpadam" vinā kārakapadam nā nvayabodham janayatīti tena tasyākāṅkṣā*. *Nyā. Sid. Muk*. p. 312-13.
4. (*a*) *arthābādho yogyatā*, *Tar. Sam*. p. 52.

(*b*) *padārthe tatra tadvattā yogyatā parikīrtitā*, *Bhā. Par kārikā*. 83.

5. *padānāmavilambena uccāranam sannidhiḥ*, *Tar. Sam*. p. 52.

6. *vṛttiśca śaktilakṣaṇānyatara sambandhaḥ*, *a Nya. Sid. Muk*. p. 264.

7. *padajñānam tu karaṇam*
dvāram tatra padārthadhīḥ|
śābdabodhaḥ phalastara
śaktidhīḥ sahakāriṇī.||
Bhā. par. (*Kārikā*,) 81.

8. See "Nature of *śabdapramāṇā*" by V.N.*Jha*, in the *Studies in Language Logic and Epistemology*.

0.4. THE CONCEPT OF *PADA*

According to the Nyāya philosophy, *śabda* is the quality of *ākāśa*. It is produced in ether. The *ākāśa* is the medium of its transmission from one place to the other. *Śabda* literally means sound. And sound is of two kinds—namely *dhvani* and *varṇa*.[1] *Dhvani* is an inarticulate sound like the sounds of drums and bells while *varṇa* is a sound produced by the vocal organ of human beings. All *varṇas* or phonemes are the constituents of human speech which are capable of forming parts of any language. Hence a word is a group of *varṇas* or phonemes, arranged in a particular order.[2]

In *Nyāya sūtra* 2.2.58 the first definition of *pada* is given by the Naiyāyikas. It is as follows : *te bibhaktyantāḥ padam*. The sequence of phonemes ending in an inflected suffix is called as *padas*. The Bhāṣyakāra elaborates *yathādarśanam vikṛtāḥ varṇāḥ vibhaktyantāḥ padasaṁjñā bhavanti.*[3] A finished form ends either in a case suffix or in a personal suffix which is called a *pada*. The *Nyāya Bhāṣya* says *vibhakir dvayaī nāmikī ākhyātikī ca*. This definition of *pada* is identical with that of Pāṇini's sūtra (1.4.14) — *suptiṅantam padam* which refers to the twofold division as— (i) those ending in a case-sufix and (ii) those ending in a personal sufiix. But the above two definitions are formal definition of a word. Uddyotakara also follows the same patteren of defining a *pada*. He says *nāmikī svādayaḥ, ākhyātikī tibādayaḥ tayā viśiṣyamāṇam padam dvedhā bhavati nāma ca ākhyātam ca*. In the *Nyāyamañjarī*, Jayanta while discussing the nature of a *śabda* defines a *pada* as a group of *varṇas* or phonemes.[4] Bhāsarvajña[5] also defines a *pada* in a similar manner.

The *Gautama Sūtravṛtti* defines in a different manner-*vṛttimattvam padatvam*[6] '*pada* is being possessed of a *vṛtti*.' *Vṛtti* is the relation between a word and its meaning. Here this definition does not give a formal definition of a word, but it is a semantic definition. It says that a meaningful unit of an expression is a *pada*.

The *Vaiśeṣika sūtropaskāra* (2.2.21) gives altogether a similar definition—*saṅketavadvarṇatvam padatvam* 'the state of being a sequence of phonemes possessing *saṅketa* is *pada*'. The term *saṅketa* means the expressive power of a word i.e. the relation between word and meaning.

Similar is the definition given by Annambhaṭṭa in his *Tarkasaṁgraha*—*śaktam padam*.[7] *Śaktam* means 'possessed of *śakti*' i.e. *śaktiviśiṣṭa padam*. A word is that which has the expressive power. According to the neo-logicians *śakti* and *saṅketa* are synonymous terms.

In *Tarkakaumudī*, Laugākṣibhāskara while discussing Verbal testimony defines a *pada* in a different manner. He says *arthavācakam padam* 'a word is that which expresses a meaning'. And also immediately he gives the two-fold division of a word-viz, primary and secondary.[8] Gokulanātha also has tried to define a *pada* in his *Padavākya ratnākara*. He says—'a state of being a *pada* is that where there is a gap of four or five moments between the earlier and the latter phoneme'.[9] But the commentator, Yadunātha Mishra defines from the standpoint of meaning. He says—*śābdabodhānukula sāmarthyavat padatvam* 'the state of being a *pada* is that which possesses the *sāmarthya* (the expressive power of a word) which is conducive of generating a verbal understanding'.

What appears from the above definitions that, *Gautamasūtravṛtti* employs a cover term *vṛtti* which stands for both the powers of words, where as *Upaskāra* and *Tarkasaṁgraha* use the particular terms (specific) *saṅketa* and *śakti* respectively. But from the use of the term *śakti and saṅketa* some one may feel that a word having secondary power *lakṣaṇā* is not a *pada*. But it is not true because unless there is *śakti* (the primary relation) there is no possibility of accepting *lakṣaṇā*—the secondary relation. *Śakti* is a necessary condition for *lakṣaṇā*. That is why *lakṣaṇā* is defined as 'the relation with the expressed sense'. So there is no difficulty in the above definition of *pada*. And taking this notion, the Naiyāyikas have given a two-fold division of *pada* namely—*mukhya* and *gauṇa*. The two types of words are further divided into different categories on the basis of the relationships. We are going to discuss in detail in the forthcoming chapters.

Another point is noteworthy here. In the beginning, the Naiyāyīkas' definition of *pada* is based on a formal aspect and not in terms of meaning whereas the later Naiyāyīkas, however defined *pada* in terms of meaning. From the above clarification of the definition of *pada*, it is clear that in *Prācīna Nyāya* the sentence *Devadaṭṭaḥ grāmam gacchati* consists of three *padas* namely—*Devadaṭṭaḥ*, *grāmam* and *gacchati*. But for the Navya Naiyāyīkas, the same expression consists of six *padas* namely—*Devadaṭṭa*, the nominative suffix—*śu*, *grāma*, the accusative suffix—*am*, the root—*gam* and the personal ending—*ti*. Thus whatever linguistic unit is meaningful is treated as *pada* according to the Neo-logicians. This notion of *pada* is identical with the notion of morpheme in Modern Linguistics.[10]

Notes

1. *śabdo dvividhaḥ dhvanyātmaka varṇātmakaśca. Dinakarī*, p. 546.
2. *padam ca varṇasamuhaḥ Tar. Bhā.* p. 126.
3. *Nyā. Bhā.* on 2.2.58.
4. *kim punaridam padam nāma, kim ca vākyamiti, uktamatra varṇa-samūhaḥ padam, padasamūho vākyamiti, Nyā Mañ*, vol. II, p. 143.
5. *Nyā Bhū*, p. 274.
6. Ānandashram Edition, p. 180.
7. P. 50.
8. *arthavācakam padam, taddvi-vidham-mukhya gauṇa bhedāt. Tar Kau*, p. 44.
9. *caturbhiḥ pañcabhirvāpi prāyeṇānta-ritaḥ Kṣaṇaiḥ | pūrvavarṇātparovarṇaḥ padatvam pratipadyate || Pad Ra*, p. 30.
10. See *Jha* V.N. *Studies in Language, Logic and Epistemology*. pp. 45-47.

0.5. THE CONCEPT OF *VĀKYA*

Neither Gautama nor Vātsyāyana gives us any definition of *vākya.* While discussing the seventh *padārtha avayava* 'inference-component' under the *sūtra* 1.1.1, Uddyotakara provides the definition of a sentence as—'a sentence is the means of the qualified knowledge (of the ward meanings) which is qualified by each word by the help of remembrance which is again qualified by the knowledge of the last word in comparison with the remembrance of the earlier word.'[1] That means a sentence gives rise to one qualified meaning which comes from the last words directly and which is again qualified by the remembrance of other words indirectly. Vācaspati Mishra also explains this fact clearly and finally defines—'a sentence is a collection of words which gives rise to a qualified meaning by the help of remembrance of other words'.[2] These two definitions are clearly based on semantic principles.

In *Nyāyamañjarī*[3], Jayanta while discussing the nature of *śabda*, defines a *pada* as a group of phonemes and a *vākya* as a collection of words. Bhāsarvajña[4] also follows the same way defining a *pada* and a *vākya.* These definitions are formal definitions. However in *Nyāyakośa,*[5] the earlier definition is recorded from the text *Tattvacintāmaṇi.* He records *vākyatvam ca viśiṣṭārthaparaśabdatvam* 'the sentence which causes a qualified knowledge'. This definition is clearly a semantic definition.

The definition of *vākya* given by Annambhaṭṭa is a formal

one. He defines—*padasamūho vākyam*[6] 'a collection of words is a sentence'. Laugākṣibhāskara[7] defines a sentence in a similar manner. But according to Keśava Mishra *vākyam tu ākāṅkṣā yogyatā sannidhimatām padānām samūhaḥ.*[8] Here, the factors like *ākāṅkṣā* 'expectancy', *yogyatā* 'compatibility' and *sannidhi* 'proximity' are included in the definition itself. Therefore, the words like *purūṣaḥ, gauḥ, hastī* etc. do not form a sentence. Because it is merely a collection of words but not having the other required factors mentioned above. Also the sentence like *bahninā siñcati* is only grammatically correct. But it is not enough for being called as a sentence. That is why the Naiyāyikas say that if an expression is simultaneously grammatically and semantically acceptable it is to be considered as a sentence. That is why the definition given by Keśava Mishra is accepted to be a better one. Annambhaṭṭa also mentions that *ākāṅkṣā, yogyatā* and *sannidhi* are the causes of the verbal knowledge.[9] In the text *Nyāyapradīpa*[10] we find a similar definition. By the term etc. he includes the other factors.

Notes

1. *kim punarvākyam ? pūrvapadasmṛtya-pekṣo'ntyapadapratyayaḥ smṛtyanugraheṇa pratisandhīyamāno viśeṣapratipatti heturvāyam. Nyāvār,* p. 48-49.
2. *tadevamekasmṛti.samāroheṇa ekārthāvacchedena padānām samūho vākyam. Nyā vār Tat Tikā,* p. 50.
3. *kim punaridam padam nāma, kim ca vākyamiti. Uktamatra varṇa-samūho padam padasamūho vākyamiti. Nyā mañ,* vol. II, p. 143.
4. *Nyā Bhū, p.* 274.
5. *Ibid* 730.
6. *Tar. Sam.* p. 50.
7. *Tarkau,* p. 44.
8. *Tar. Bhā.* p. 121.
9. *Tar. Sam.* p. 52.
10. P. 100.

0.6. THE CONCEPT OF *PADĀRTHA*

According to the Naiyāyikas the world is described in terms of *padārthas*, which are again divided in to *bhāva* and *abhāva* categories. But here we restrict our discussion of the concept of *padārtha* which refers to word meanings in the process of verbal understanding.

For verbal understanding the Naiyāyikas follow a process. This process has been explained earlier. The term *padārtha* means—*padasyārthaḥ* i.e. the meaning of the words. In a sentence there are many words. Those words have certain meanings which denote its reference. When a word is uttered in a sentence, the listener remembers the menaing of that particular word at that moment. Thus each word meaning is remembered by the listener from each word. This is called *padārtha* the word meanings of a sentence. These word meanings refer to some object (referent) which comes from the word directly or indirectly. That is why in a sentence the *śabdāhdyāhāra* is to be made according to the Naiyāyikas. But the Prābhākara Mīmāṁsakas say that—there one supplies the meaning in a sentence even though word is absent. They accept *arthādhyāhāra*, which is cumbersome for the Naiyāyikas. In the first stage the listener listens to a sentence carefully and then he slowly knows the elements of that sentence. To give an example—*Rāmaḥ tanḍulam pacati* here there are six constituents of this sentence. They are (1) *Rāma* (2) the nominative suffix (3) *tanḍula* (Rice) (4) the accusative suffix (5) the root—*gam* and

(6) the personal ending—*ti*. In this stage the knowledge of the constituents occur—

Ist stage :

Rāma— *ḥ* + *taṇḍula*—*m* + *pac*—*ti*
(1) (2) (3) (4) (5) (6)

In the next stage—the listener remembers the word meanings from the respective words of the sentence uttered.

Ist stage.	*Rāma*	— *ḥ* +	*taṇḍula*—*m*	+	*pac* —	*ti*
	(1)	(2)	(3)	(4)	(5)	(6)
IInd stage.	*Rāma*	Singular number etc.	rice	objectness	to cook	volition (present tense)
	(1)	(2)	(3)	(4)	(5)	(6)

In this second stage 1, 2, 3, 4, 5 and 6 are treated as *padārthas*.

0.7. THE CONCEPT OF *VĀKYĀRTHA*

As we have discussed that the verbal understanding has a process which follows some stages. When the listener listens to a sentence he at first knows the individual constituents of the sentence. Here in this stage—(1)

Rāma	—	*ḥ*	*grāma*	—	*m*	*gaccha*	*ti*
(1)		(2)	(3)		(4)	(5)	(6)

(1), (2), (3), (4), (5), and (6) are called *padas.* After the *padas* are known he remembers the concerned meanings. Here in this stage—2nd

Ramā, singular number, *grāma*, objectness, act of going and volition are called *padārthas.* And in the next stage—3rd when the *padārthas* are linked to one another by a relationship these connections are called *vākyārthas.*

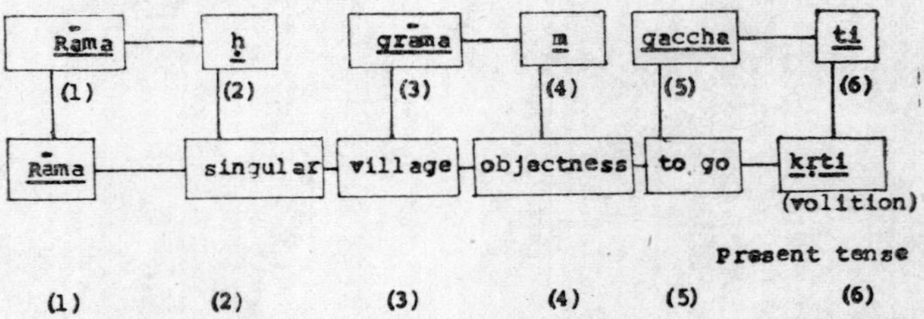

These horizontal lines which connect the *padārthas* are called *vākyārthas. Vākyārthajñāna* is that 'the knowledge referring to the relation between each word meanings of a sentence (*ekapadārthe aparapadārtha saṁsarga viṣayakajñānam*'.

0.8. THE CONCEPT OF *ŚĀBDABODHA*

The Indian Philosophical tradition provides a method of understanding a sentence. The understanding of the meaning of a sentence is known as *śābdabodha.* It is regarded as one of the four valid cognitions in Nyāya system. When a speaker utters a sentence the hearer listens to it and a communicative method is adopted to get the verbal understanding. What is this method of understanding the meaning of a sentence ? The Indian Philosophers assume a process. When the sentence is uttered the listener listens to that sentence and he tries to know the individual constituents of that sentence. This is the first stage. In the next stage he remembers the word meanings from the concerned words. After that the knowledge of the meanings are conected with each other which is the *vākyārtha* stage. After that all meanings are related together to get a whole meaning of the sentence. This is the fourth stage at which we get the knowledge of the meaning of that sentence which is called *śābdabodha.*

It has been defined as 'the knowledge caused by the efficient instrumentality of the knowledge of words' (*padajñāna karaṇakam jñānam*).[1] In other words it is defined as—'the knowledge resulting from the remembrance of meanings which is also produced by the words' (*padajanya padārthopasthitijanyabodhaḥ*). *Sābdabodha* is the final result of the process of verbal understanding. Visvanātha Nyāyapañcānana mentions that the knowledge of the words is the instrument (*karaṇa*), the knowledge of the *padārthas* is the *vyāpāra* or *dvāra* and the verbal understanding is the final result and the knowledge of *śakti* is an auxiliary factor.[2]

[*padajñāna*	...	*padārthasmaraṇa*]	→	*śābdabodha*
(*karaṇa*)	*sakti* or *lakṣaṇa*	(*dvāra* or *vyāpāra*)		(*phala*)

When the listener listens to the sentence uttered, the meaning of the constituent words is not the only condition for verbal understanding. It is no doubt the primary condition. But there are also some secondary or auxiliary conditions. For instance, in the sentence—*Rāmaḥ grāmam gacchati*, the words are known first then its expressive power (*śakti*) and both these taking together the remembrance of the meaning becomes possible. Let us analyse the sentence—*Rāmāḥ grāmam gacchati.*

Here in this sentence there are six meaningful units or words. (1) *Rāma* (2) *-aḥ* (3) *grāma* (4) *-am* (5) the root—*gam* and (6) the suffix—*ti.*

In the next stage their expressive powers are comprehended in the following manner :

The word (1) *Rāma* denotes a person Rama, (2) the nominative suffix *-aḥ* (*su*) expresses number (*prathamā* etc.), (3) the word *grāma* denotes village, (4) the accusative suffix *-am* denotes objectness (*karmatva*), (5) the root—*gam* denotes action of going, and (6) the personal suffix *ti*—expresses volition *kṛti* or *yatna* in addition to the meanings of present tense and number etc.

Not only the above relation or expressive power (*śakti*) is enough but also the factors like *ākāṅkṣā*, *yogyatā*, *sannidhi* and *tātparya* are the auxiliary conditions for the production of *śābdabodha.*

According to the Indian thinkers and linguists there are three ways of understanding a sentence. By this we refer to the Mimāṁsakas, the Naiyāyikas and the Grammarians. The Mimāṁsakas say that—the process we follow for *śābdabodha* is based on where the meaning of the personal suffix is the prime qualificand (*ākhyātārthamukhyaviśeṣyaka-śābdabodhaḥ*).

The Naiyāyikas accept the *śābdabodha* where the meaning of the noun in the nominative case is the prime qualificand (*prathamāntārthamukhya-viśeṣyaka-śābdabodhaḥ*).

And the Grammarians accept that the meaning of the verbal root is the prime qualificand (*dhātvartha-mukhya-viśeṣyaka śābdabodhaḥ*).

Now I restrict my discussion only to the Naiyāyikas way of analysing the knowledge of sentence meaning. In the earlier sentence—*Rāmaḥ grāmam gacchati*, here we have analysed the words earlier. Here in this sentence *Rāma* is the prime qualificand (*mukhya viśeṣya*) and the rest of it is only the *prakāra* 'qualifier'. All the words are correlated to one part or the other in a definite order. That means there is a relation of qualifier and qualificand in the sentence. Thus here in the sentence—the meaning is that of the prime qualificand *Rāma* qualified by the action conducive to the contact with the subsequent place having *grāma* as its object (*grāmakarmakagamanānukula prakāraka kṛtimān Rāmāḥ* or *grāmagamanānukula kṛtimān Rāmaḥ*).

This understanding can be explained in the following manner. Here there are six elements.

[(1) — 2 — 3 — 4 — 5 — 6]

mukha-viśeṣya   *prakāra*

In the case—

[(2) — 3 — 4 — 5 — 6]

mukhya-viśeṣya   *Prakāra*

And this kind of connection or relationship follows one after the other. But the fact is that (1) always remains as the prime qualificand (*mukhya-viśeṣya*)—even though in the subsequent stages the qualifier and qualificand change. Hence those remembered meanings form one integrated structure of the qualifier and qualificand type. This knowledge is what is called the *śābdabodha.*

If someone asks that how do you get the relations (horizontal lines in the structure 1......... 2,......... 3,......... 4, ... 5, ...6). In this regard there are a number of opinions. The Bhāṭṭas hold that it is possible to get the integrated meanings through *lakṣaṇā*, the Prābhākaras say through the constituent elements of the sentence—1, 2, 3, 4, 5 and 6. But the Naiyāyikas say—that those are obtained by the help of *Saṁsargamaryādā* or juxtaposition. For this issue the Bhāṭṭas advocate the theory of *Abhihitānvayavāda*, the Prābhākaras propose the theory of *Anvitābhidhānavāda* and the Naiyāyikas say that it is the *saṁsargamaryādāvāda.*

Notes

1. *vākyārthajñānam śābdajñānam*, *Tar. Saṁ.* p. 54.
2. *Padajñānam tu karaṇam dvāram tatra padārthadhīḥ/ śābdabodhaḥ phalastatra śaktidhīḥ sahakāriṇi//* *Bhā. Par.* (*Kārikā*), p. 81.

1.0. CLASSIFICATION OF WORDS

Various parameters can be applied for the classification of word. Yāska the famous grammarian and etymologist classifies words in to four classes namely—noun, verb, prepositions and indeclinables. He mentions thus in *Nirukta—tad yāni catvāri padajātāni nāmākhyāte copasarganipātāśca tānīmāni bhavanti.*

Pāṇini broadly classifies words into two groups.[1] They are (i) *subanta*—words ending in a case suffix and (ii) *tiṅanta*—words ending in a personal suffix. That means a *pada* is that which ends either in a case suffix or a personal suffix.

Patañjali however, supplies two fold classification of words in Sanskrit language namely—the ordinary words—*laukika śabda* and the scriptural words—*vaidika śabda*. This is a kind of classification of words from cultural point of view. He gives examples for these two types of classification of words. The *laukika śabdas* are like *gauḥ* 'cow', *aśvaḥ* 'horse', *puruṣa* 'man', *hasti* 'elephant' and the like. So also the *vaidika śabdas* are as follows—*saṅnodevīrabhiṣṭaye, agnīmīḷe purohitam* and the like. He mentions in the following manner :—*keṣām śabdānām laukikānām vaidikānām ca. tatra laukikāstāvad goraśva puruṣo hastī śakunirmṛgo brāhmaṇa iti, vaidikāḥ khalvapi saṅnodevīrabhiṣṭaye* (*Ma. Bhā.* on 1.1.1). Patañjali does not stop here. He also records the four-fold classification as given by Yāska.[2] He also has *jāti, guṇa, kriyā* and *yadṛcchā śabdas*.

Gautama and Vātsyāyana too mention the two-fold classification of words as *dṛṣṭārtha* i.e. *laukika* and *adṛṣṭārtha* i.e. *vaidika*.[3] *Dṛṣṭārtha* is that what is related to the perceptible objects and *adṛṣṭārtha* is that which is related to the imperceptible objects. The first category applies to the expressions of ordinary earthly sensible objects uttered by the trustworthy persons. Where as the second division is applied to the expressions or usages of super-sensible objects like *aṇu, paramāṇu, dharma, pāpa, puṇya* and *mokṣa* etc. informed by the prophets or saints.

Jaimini however, in the second chapter of the *Mīmāṁsā sūtras* defines only two classes of words namely—*Karmaśabdaḥ* and *nāmāni.* He defines *nāmāni*[4] as words on the utterance of which the forms of the objects denoted by them become apprehended. In other words he says that *nāmāni* are the names of some accomplished objects. But *karmaśabdas*[5] denote something which is yet to be accomplished.

Where as Śabara goes further and include substance and adjective in *nāmāni.* He paraphrases the word *nāmāni* by *dravya guṇa śabdāḥ.*[6] Besides that Śabara has also given us one more class of words namely the *sarvanāman* which Jaimini does not seem to have expressly mentioned.

So we can say that according to Jaimini and Śabara there are two and four different classes of words respectively namely—*nāma, ākhyāta* or *karmaśabda, sarvanāma* and *viśeṣaṇa.*

When the words are classified on the parameters of relation between a word and its meaning, we get such classification as *yaugika, rūḍha, yogarūḍha* and *yaugikarūḍha.*

Notes

1. *subtiṅantam padam.*
2. *catvāri vākparimītā padāni, catvāri padajātāni nāmākhyātopasarganipātāśca. Ma. Bhā.* (*Pasp.*) on 1.1.1.
3. *sa dvividho dṛṣṭādṛṣṭārthatvāt. Nyā. Sū.* 1.1.8. and *Bhā.*

4. *yeṣāmutpattau sve prayoge rūṇopalabdhistāni nāmāni. Mīm. Sū.* II. 1.3.
5. (*i*) *bhāvārthāḥ karmaśabdāḥ*, Ibid. II. 1.1.
   (*ii*) *yeṣām tutpattāvarthe sve prayogo na vidyate tānyākhyātāni* Ibid. II. 1.4.
6. *te dravyaguṇaśabdā iti vaktavya tāni nāmānīti sūtritam, yato nāmānītyeṣām paryāyaśabdaḥ, Śāb. Bhā.* p. 387.

1.1. TYPES OF WORDS

In Sanskrit there are two types of stems namely (i) nominal stems and (ii) verbal stems. When suffixes are added to them they appear in finished form.

Patañjali in his *Mahābhāṣya* refers to three kinds of words. They are (i) *sādhu śabdas* (ii) *apaśabdaś* and (iii) *apabhraṁśas*. He claims that one who knows the correct words knows also incorrect words. And as a result of which merit (*dharma*) follows from the utterance of correct words and demerit (*adharma*) from the incorrect words.[1] He says that there are many incorrect words and less correct words. Each and every word has many *apabhraṁśas* which are pronounced differently.[2]

He does not stop here. He again divides words in a different manner into four categories. They are *jātiśabda*, *guṇaśabda*, *krīyāśabda* and *yadṛcchāśabdas*.[3] He also supplies sufficient examples for each of these categories. He mentions—*goḥ śukla-ścalo ḍitthaḥ ityādau catuṣṭayī śabdānām prvṛttiriti*. This division is based on the nature of words.

We find another kind of division of words namely (i) *tatsama* (ii) *tadbhava* and (iii) *deśaja*. *Tatsama* is that which is quite similar to that of Sanskrit, *Tadbhava* is that which is derived from Sanskrit and *Deśaja* words are purely of native origin.

It is also a fact that for some words etymology can be given and for some it cannot be. That means some words are derivable and some are not. But the etymologist grammarian Śākaṭāyana hold the view that all nouns are derived from verbal roots. Following is the statement: *nāmāni ākhyātajānīti śākaṭāyano nairuktasamayaśca.* But the other grammarian namely Gārgya opposes the above statement. He claims that there are some nouns which cannot be derived. The statement runs as under—

na sarvāṇīti gārgyo vaiyākaraṇānāmcaike. Those are called underivable stems. Such words can be called *avyutpanna prātipadikas* (underivable stems). These are brought under *uṇādi* rules.

The Mīmāṁsakas have the following division of words.

(1) *Jātiśabda*

The words which are found to denote *jati* in one place must denote in all places. Such words are called *jātinimittāḥ śabdāḥ* or *jātiśabdāḥ* in Mimāṁsā system. The word *varhiḥ* for example is used as a *jātiśabda* without any reference to any *sāṁskāra.* The word refers to a variety of grass. But the problem is whether it is a *jātiśabda* or a *saṁskāra śabda*? They answer that the word is known as a *jātiśabda* because *jāti* is found to be the *pravṛttinimitta* of a *śabda.*[4]

(2) *Saṁskāra Sabda*

The words which are used on a particular *saṁskāra* which have to be performed on that occasion are called as *saṁskāra śabdas.* For example the word *yūpa* will not be used at all if the particular *saṁskāras* are not performed over the sacrificial post. *Saṁskāra,* therefore, is accepted as the *pravṛttinimitta* of the word *yūpa* and hence the word *yūpa* is termed as *saṁskāra śabda.*

(3) *Yaugika*

The words when come to usage not directly by its own meaning, but by some connection (*yoga* or *saṁyoga*) with some other word already in usage, such words are called *yaugika* or *yoga-siddha.* For example the word *rājya* depends for its currency (*prasiddhi*) on the word *rājan.* The word *rājan* is the *prasiddhimūla.* Śabara rightly points out that, *Rājaśabdaḥ prasiddher mūlam, tadyogād rājyaśabdaḥ.*[5] Here such words have *yoga* 'connection or association' as *pravṛttinimitta*. The word *rājan* is a *jātiśabda* and serves as the basis for the currency (*prasiddhimūla*) of the word *rājya*.

(4) *Sambandhī Śabda*

The words which are related to some other word by which the word can only come in to existence is called *Sambandhi Śabda*. For example, the word *putra* depends for its *prasiddhi* on *sambandha* of the person with his father. It suggests that the word *putra* can be used with reference to a person only if he is connected with another person as his son. It is also the same case with the word *pitṛ*. Both these words *putra* and *pitṛ* are mutually dependent and hence called *sambandhi śabdas*. Śabara writes : *sambandhi śabdaśca sarve sāpekṣā vinā padāntareṇa na paripūrṇam artham abhivadanti.*[6]

(5) *Rūḍha śabda*

According to the Mīmāṁsakas this is another types of *śabda*, where *rūḍhi* serves as the *pravṛttinimitta*. For example : the word *kuśala* if taken etymologically, means 'one who cuts kuśa grass' and by indication (*lakṣaṇā*) it may denote all the qualities which express excellence or skill. But this skilfulness is the meaning prevalent in the usage. The secondary meaning i.e. skilfulness has restricted the possibility of the application of etymological sense. And hence the word *kuśala* means *nīpuṇatā*. According to Śabara[7] the meaning *nīpuṇatā* is the *vācyārtha* of the word *kuśala*. Here the *pravṛttinimitta* of the word *kuśala* and *pravīṇa* is *rūḍhi*. The Mīmāṁsakas say that—when there are two meanings possible of a word, there *rūḍhi* is predominant, Here the same example is given and for this they have a rule that—the etymological sense is always weaker than the conventional sense i.e. *avayavaprasiddher samudāyaprasiddhir valīyasī*.

According to the Naiyāyikas, the word is capable of expressing two meanings. One is direct or primary and another is indirect or secondary or implied. Therefore, *vṛtti*, through which a word refers to something is twofold—(i) *śakti*—the primary relation and (ii) *Lakṣaṇā*—the secondary relation. The first is operative with the desire (*śakti* or *saṅketa*) and the second one entirely is dependent on *śakti*. That is why *lakṣaṇā* is defined as connection with the primary meaning. According to the definition *śaktam padam*, *śaktam* also accommodates *lākṣaṇika śabda*. Unless a *pada* is *śakta* it cannot be *lākṣaṇika*. There is also another division of words namely—*pāribhāṣika pada*[8]. This category refer to the technical words like *nadī*, *guṇa*, *vṛddhi*, *ghu* etc. which are the creations of the *śāstrakāras*.

Then comes the four types of words namely—(i) *yaugika* 'etymological or derivative' (ii) *rūḍha* 'conventional' (iii) *yoga-rūḍha* 'etymologico-conventional or derivative-conventional' and (iv) *yaugika—rūḍha* 'both etymological and conventional, which come under *śakta* category. These words are discussed individually in the following chapter.

Notes

1. *yo hi śabdān jānāti apaśabdānapyasau jānāti, yathaiva hi śabdajñāne dharmaḥ evam apaśabdajñāne'pi adharmaḥ. Ma. Bhā.* 1.1.1.
2. *bhūyāṁso'paśabdāḥ alpiyāṁsaḥ śabdāḥ, ekaikasya hi śabdasya bahavo'pabhraṁśāḥ.* Ibid.
3. *catuṣṭayi sabdānām pravṛttiḥ, jātiśabdāḥ, guṇaśabdāḥ kriyāśabdāḥ yadṛcchāśabdāścaturthāḥ. Ma. Bhā.* 1.1.2.
4. *Śāb. Bhā. on Mīm. Sū.* I. 4.10.
5. Ibid. II. 3.3.
6. *Mim. Sū.*—VI. 7.24.
7. *Sāb. Bhā. on Mim. Sū.* VI. 7.21-22.
8. *tatrādhunikasaṅketaḥ paribhāṣā tayā cārthabodhakam padam pāribhāṣikam yathā śāstrakārādiśaṅketita nadī vṛddhyādi padam. Śakti.* p. 5.

1.1.1. *YAUGIKA, RŪḌHA, YOGARŪḌHA* AND *YAUGIKARŪḌHA**

In Navya-Nyāya system of Philosophy, the words are generally divided into four classes namely—(i) *Yaugika* 'etymological', (ii) *Rūḍha* 'conventional' (iii) *Yogarūḍha* 'etymologico-conventional' and (iv) *Yaugikarūḍha* sometimes 'both which could be taken either as etymological or as conventional'.[1] These four categories of words are divided according to different ways in which their meanings are determined on the basis of the expressive relation of a word. A detailed discussion follows on each category of words.

Each word has certain meaning and it stands for something which is referred to by that word. That is called as word-meaning or the object of reference of that word. But naturally the question arises how the words convey the objects? The following answer is given. It is because of the relationship existing between the word and its referent i.e. *vṛtti*[2] that a word conveys a meaning. This relationship can be either primary or secondary.

(1) *Yaugika*

The meaning of a *Yaugika śabda* is determined by the expressive meaning of its component parts.[3] For example, the word *pācaka* 'cook.' Here the meaning of this word is known

*See *Dash*, S.C, 'Śaśadhara's arguments in favour of *Yogarūḍhi*' *JOIB*, Vol. 37. 3-4, pp. 333-38.

from the verbal root *pac* 'to cook' and the suffix—*aka* signifying the agent of the action of cooking. Such words are derived words, that is why it is called etymological words. In such cases grammar helps a lot to decide the meaning through primary relation. The root meaning and the meaning of suffix are taken into consideration for deciding the meaning as a whole. The compound words like *ratha-kāra* 'one who makes a chariot', *ghaṭakāra* 'one who makes a pot' also fall under this category. Such words consist of two members namely—*ratha* and *kāra*, *ghaṭa* and *kāra* and their meanings are determined by the help of the individual meanings of the two members (*avayavas*). That is the reason that the Naiyāyikas do not accept a separate *śakti* called *Śamāsaśakti*. Here the *yogaja śakti* or *yoga* determines the meaning.

(2) *Rūḍha*

A word is called *rūḍha* 'conventional' when it has a meaning which is not directly connected with its etymological meaning. In this case, the meaning is determined by the conventional usage. The term *rūḍhi* is defined as 'the expressive relation in the whole word without any reference to its parts.[4] In other words when a particular sense is conveyed by a particular word from time immemorial it is said that, the word is conventionally used in that sense. The words like *gauḥ* 'cow', *ghaṭaḥ* 'pot,' *paṭaḥ* 'cloth' are used conventionally to refer to those objects or entities. Underivable simple words called *avyutpannas* belong to this category. For example, the words like, *go*, *ghaṭa*, *paṭa* etc. are treated as conventional words. It can be said that the words whose etymology is not transparent and whose origin is not known are the *rūḍha* words.

(3) *Yogarūḍha*

When a word is found to be used in a conventional sense to which the etymological sense also applies it is called *Yogarūḍha*[5] 'etymologico-conventional or derivative-conventional' type of words. This is the third category of words in which the word has a conventional meaning which coincides with the etymological meaning. The word *paṅkaja* is widely accepted as lotus by convention but at the same time the etymological sense is also applicable to it. By the acceptance of the conventional sense, the etymological sense is completely restricted. Otherwise, the term *paṅkaja* might mean anything which grows in the mud like frog, lily and moss etc. It is our normal experience that, when anyone listens to the word *paṅkaja*, the conventional sense comes to his mind and the meaning lotus is remembered by him and not the etymological sense. In other words, we can say that the conventional sense predominates over the etymological sense.

That is why there is a well known rule accepted by the Indian Philosophers. It says that the conventional meaning is more powerful than the etymological meaning (*yogād rūḍhir-valiyasī śīghravṛttitvāt*). It is because the former occurs to the mind quickly whereas the latter has to be known through proper analysis of the grammatical rules.

The word *paṅkaja* is derived from the word *paṅka* (mud) and *ja* (born of). Etymologically, the word means that which grows in the mud. But as a matter of fact, the literal meaning is not taken into consideration here. Thus, it is called partly etymological and partly conventional. There are various examples for this class of words of which the famous word is *kṛṣṇasarpa*, which etymologically means—'black-snake', but the conventional usage of this word is with reference to the poisonous 'cobra' only.[6]

Such words are not only used in Sanskrit Literature, but also in the English Literature. For example, the word 'morning-star' which is restricted only to a particular star that is visible in the morning and does not refer to any other star which are visible in the morning.

(4) *Yaugikarūḍha*

When a word is found used in both etymological as well as conventional sense, is it called *yaugikarūḍha* 'etymological and conventional' type of words.[7] The meaning is determined either etymologically from the meanings of the components or conventionally from the usage of the whole word. As the example given – *udbhid* etc., which is used in the sense of a 'sprout,' when considered in its etymological sense, but when it is used in the sense of 'sacrifice,' one must say that it is used in a conventional sense. Both the meanings are determined independently of each other and hence understood in separate contexts. This category of words often referred to as *rūḍhayaugika.* Take another example—*aśvagandhā* is a complex word which consists of the word *aśva* (horse) and *gandhā* (smell). It etymologically means—'that which smells like a horse.' But the very word denotes a medicinal herb mentioned in *Āyurveda,* which has nothing to do with a horse or its smell. This word is an instance of two words with two different meanings having the same form, one being *yaugika* (*gandhā*) and the other *rūḍha* (*aśva*). Both the meanings are conveyed by the same word independently with different contexts.

This categorization is dependent on the four fold divisions of *śakti* namely—(i) *yoga* (ii) *rūḍhi* (iii) *yogarūḍhi* and (iv) *yaugikarūḍhi.* It seems that the Naiyāyikas are very logical while deciding the meaning of words on the basis of the expressive relation. Another point is to be noted that, the relations are the deciding factors while interpreting the word meanings in Nyāya system.

Notes

1. *śaktam padam tu kvaciddyaugikam, kvacidrūḍham, kvacidyogarūḍham, kvacidyaugikarūḍham. Nyā. Si. Muk.* p. 282.

2. *vṛttirnāma śaktilakṣaṇānyatararūpā. Nyā. Bo.* p. 52.

3. (i) *avayavaśakitryogaḥ. Tar. Dīp.* p. 51.

   (ii) *yatrāvayavārtha eva budhyate taddyaugikam, Nyā. Si. Muk.* p. 282.

4. (i) *samudāyaśaktirrūḍhiḥ*. *Tar. Dīp.* p. 51.
   (ii) *yatrāvayavaśaktinirapekṣayā samudāyaśaktyā budhyate tadrūḍham*. *Nyā. Si. Muk.* p. 283.
5. (i) *yatra tu avayavaśaktiviṣaye samudāya-śaktirapyasti tadyogarūḍham*. *Nyā. Si. Muk.* p. 283.
   (ii) *yogena sahitā rūḍhiriti*. *Nīlakaṇṭhī*. 4.31.
6. *yan nāma svāvayava vṛtti labhyārthena samam svārthasyānvayavodhakṛt, tan nāma yogarūḍham yathā paṅkaja kṛṣṇasarpādharmādi*. *Śab. Śa. Pra.* p. 160.
7. *yadi tu yaugikārtha rūḍhyarthayoḥ svātantryeṇabodhastaddyaugikarūḍham, yathodbhidādipadam*. *Nyā. Si. Muk.* p. 285.

2.0. CONCEPT OF *SĀMARTHYA*

The word *sāmarthya* is a synonym of *śakti*. The problem arises when there is a complex form, how to get the meaning ? Is it a single unit and the meaning is known from that or the meaning is determined by the relationships of the constituents of the complex form. In other words whether there is no necessity of postulating such a relationship with the compound as a whole (single unit) and the primary relationships of the constituents of a compound with their individual meanings will take care of the meaning of the complex form ? This is the dialogue between the Grammarians and the Naiyāyikas. The Grammarians say it is necessary to postulate an additional relationship called *sāmarthya* in the compound form as a whole over and above the relationships of the constituents of that compound.

Pāṇini 2.1.1. (*Samarthaḥ padavidhiḥ*) records in his *Aṣṭādhyāyī* the concept of *samartha* which means semantically connected'. The rule as a whole means that wherever a grammatical operation concerning finished form is prescribed, it must be applied to words which are semantically connected. This *sāmārthya*[1] is of two types namely : (1) *Ekārthībhāva* and *vyapekṣā*. But Patañjali says that *sāmarthya* is the 'semantic connection', which should be understood in the sense of *ekārthībhāva* i.e. single-integrated meaning. The division of *sāmarthya* in to *ekārthībhāvaḥ* and *vyapekṣā* is not known explicitly or implicitly to Pāṇini. These two interpretations of *sāmarthya* developed from the time of Kātyāyana.[2] This statement needs re-examination. It is true that in these very two terms Pāṇini does not mention *sāmarthya*. But whether these cannot be implied even, needs to be gone into.

Notes

1. See *Jha*, V.N. 'On *Ekārthībhāva* and *Vyapekṣā*,' Studies in Language Logic and Epistemology, pp. 54-69.
2. See *Joshi*, S.D. *Samarthāhnika*.

2.1. CONCEPT OF *EKĀRTHĪBHĀVA*

Over the issue whether there should be an additional relationship over and above the relationships of the constituents of the compound with their meanings or there is no necessity of accepting it, the Grammarians reply that—yes we have the necessity of postulating an additional relationship *sāmarthya* in the compound form. Even though the relationships of the constituents of that compound is present. This expressive capacity or relationship is called *ekārthībhāva*—'emergence of single integrated meaning.'

For example in the compound *rājapuruṣaḥ*, there are two *padas* namely—*rājan* and *puruṣaḥ*. We can have another form conveying the same sense *rājñāḥpuruṣaḥ* as conveyed by the word *rājapuruṣaḥ*. But there is a little difference between these two. The genetive ending (*-as*) expresses the relation between the king and the man in the case of *rājñaḥ puruṣaḥ*. But also the same relationship is expressed in the other case where there is no—*as* genetive suffix of the word *rājapuruṣaḥ*. That is why to get the meaning of the deleted—*as* suffix the Grammarians postulate *ekārthībhāva sāmarthya* in the whole compound word *rāja-puruṣaḥ*. But the Naiyāyikas don't accept this. They define *ekārthībhāva* as—*viśeṣya—viśeṣaṇa bhāvāvagāhi ekopasthitijanakatvam*[1] i.e.—being the producer of a remembrance in which the meanings of a complex formation appear as qualifier-qualificand. Kaiyaṭa however defines—*ekārthībhāva* as that where the constituent words (of a compound) the meanings of which have been subordinated or which have lost their own meanings or which have become redundant because of adopting the prime sense or which convey a sense other than their own sense (*yatra padāni upasarjani-bhūtasvārthāni nivṛttasvārthāni vā pradhānārthopādānāt vyarthāni arthāntarābhidhāyinī vā sa ekārthi-bhāvaḥ*).[2]

Notes

1. *Nyā. Ko.* p. 771.
2. See *Joshi*, S.D. *Vyākaraṇa Mahābhāṣya* (*Samarthāhnika*) pp. 8-9.

2.2. CONCEPT OF *VYAPEKṢĀ*

The Grammarians accept *ekārthībhāva* a special relation on the compound over and above the relationships of the constituents of that compound. In the compound *rājapuruṣaḥ*, the relation expresses the meaning as a whole *rājasambandhī puruṣaḥ* through *ekārthībhāva.*

But the Naiyāyikas on the otherhand refute this above proposal and maintain that, the expressive powers of the constituents of a compound are capable enough to express the compound meaning. This individual capacity of each constituent of a compound conveys meaning and through the mutual expectancy the compound-meaning is known. This is what is called as *vyapekṣā.*

The definition as recorded in the *Nyāyakoṣa*[1] as *parasparanirūpyanirūpakabhāvāpanna viṣayatāprayojakatve sati ekārthopasthityajanakatvam* 'being the prompter of the *viṣayatās* which are mutually describer of each other and at the same time not being the producer of the remembrance of single integrated meaning'. Kaiyaṭa defines *vyapekṣā* as *parasparākāṅkṣārūpā vyapekṣā* i.e. *vyapekṣa* is of the form of mutual expectancy (between two words conveying their meanings separately).[2]

The Naiyāyikas argue that in the case of the compound *rājapuruṣaḥ* no extra relationship is needed. If the words *rājā* can express *rājasambandhin* and if *puruṣa* can express 'man' then it is clear that the compound *rājapuruṣaḥ* conveys *rājasambandhī puruṣaḥ*—because it is logically simpler. And if it is asked how the word *sambadhin* appear from the word *rājā*. We say it is by *lakṣaṇā* we obtain the meaning *rājasambandhin*.

Difference between the two

Patañjali refers to *sāmarthya* and says—it is of two types—(i) *vyapekṣā* and (ii) *ekārthībhāva*. *Vyapekṣā* i.e. interdependence of meaning exists only in groups of uncompounded words like *rājñaḥ puruṣaḥ* 'kings man'. In this example the words depend on one another to make the meaning syntactically complete. But single integrated meaning i.e. *ekārthībhāva* exists only in the integrated forms like *rājapuruṣaḥ* 'king-man'. In the case of the uncompounded word-group, the word meanings are presented separately by the stems which are linked together by one relation indicated by the inflected suffixes. But in the case of a compound, the meaning is not presented by the constituent words and of their relation existing between them. The compound as a whole denotes a single meaning in which the grammatical relation between the constituents also obtain 'the status of a word-meaning'.

The difference between *ekārthībhāva* and *vyāpekṣā* which determines the nature of an uncompounded expression and a compound form, is based on the manner of presentation of the meaning. The two expressions *rājapuruṣaḥ* and *rājñapuruṣaḥ* have almost identical meaning and refer to one and the same person.

Notes

1. p. 971.
2. See *Jha* V.N. Studies in Language Logic and Epistemology p. 54-69.

3.0. RELATION BETWEEN WORD AND ITS MEANING

In the process of verbal understanding when the words are uttered and the listener listens to those words, at that time he is reminded of the respective meanings of those words. This remembrance of meaning is possible through the relationship existing between them. That relation is called *vṛtti* i.e. the expressive relation of a word. The knowledge of that relation is very important in the context of the process of verbal understanding. It is defined as the relationship existing between the word and its meaning which is capable of generating the remembrance of the word meaning which is essential for the verbal understanding.[1]

This *vṛtti*[2] is divided into two categories namely *śakti* and *lakṣaṇā*. *Śakti* is the primary relation and *lakṣaṇā* is the secondary relation between the word and its meaning. In other words these primary and secondary relations are commonly known by the term *vṛtti*. The Grammarians also accept *vṛtti* as a relation between word and its meaning which generates verbal understanding.[3] The words like *samaya*[4] and *sāmarthya*[5] were used instead of *śakti* as the word meaning relation in *prācīna Nyāya*.

3.1. *ŚAKTI*

Śakti is one of the relations used for verbal understanding. It is the primary relation which generates the remembrance of word-meanings from words. Without the knowledge of a relation, the *śābdabodha* does not arise at all. That is why the definition says—*śakti* is regarded as a relation between the word and its meaning.[6] It is of the form of God's desire such as from such a word such meaning is to be understood.[7] According to the Neo-logicians, *śakti* and *saṅketa* are synonymous terms. But *saṅketa* is not only to be accepted as *Īśvarecchā* but also the desire of man. So *saṅketa* 'desire' is divided in to two categories :

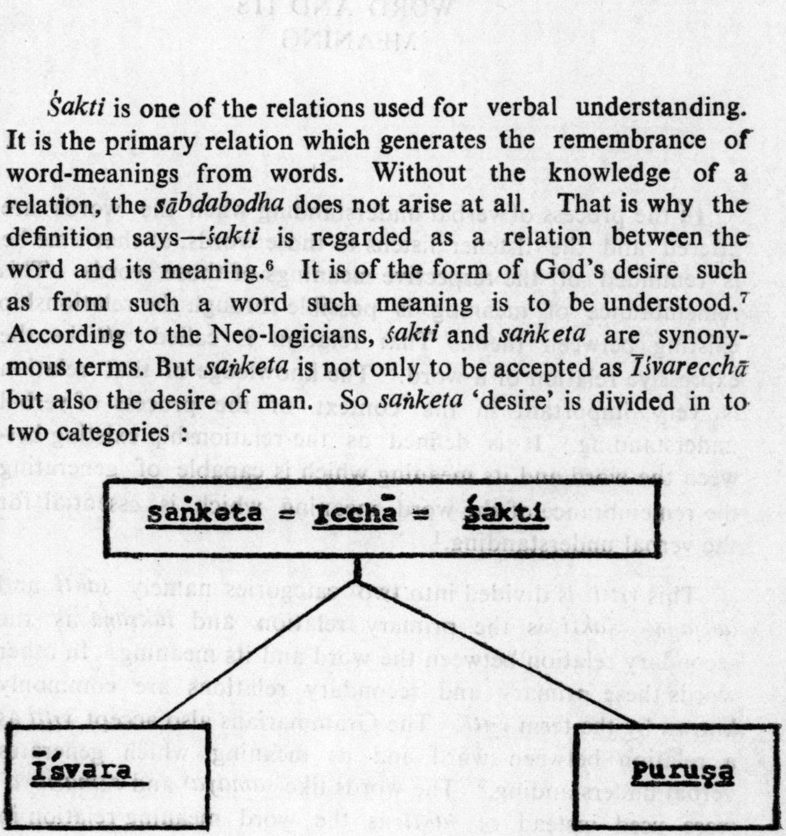

Gadādhara refers to the *ādhunika śaṅketa* which is man's creation and words having *ādhunika śaṅketa* are called the technical terms (*pāribhāṣika śabdas*) : for example the terms like—*guṇa vṛddhi, nadī* etc.[8]

But the Neo-logicians accept that not only the desire of God, even man's desire should be treated as *śakti* of a word.[9] The Naiyāyikas accept four kinds of *śakti* namely : (i) *yoga* (ii) *rūḍhi* (iii) *yogarūḍhi* and (iv) *yaugikarūḍhi*. Let us analyse them one by one.

(i) *Yoga*

Yoga is defined as the capacity of generating the meaning from the union of the meanings of parts or components of a word.[10] For example, the word *pācaka* is divided in to two parts (i) the root *pac* 'to cook' and (ii) the suffix *aka* refers to the agency. Then after joining together the meaning 'one who cooks' we get the whole meaning of the term *pācaka*. And hence the corresponding words are called *yaugikas* which are derivable.

(ii) *Rūḍhi*

It is defined as 'the expressive relation in the whole word without any reference to its parts.[11] The examples are *go, hastī, puruṣa, aśva, ghaṭa* and *paṭa* etc. The *samudāyaśakti* applies to the whole word and the meaning are remembered. The corresponding words are called *rūḍha*.

(iii) *Yogarūḍhi*

This is the third type of relation where both etymological as well as conventional meanings are considered.[12] This kind of *śakti* restricts the application of *avayavaśakti* and hence the conventional sense predominates over *avayavaśakti*. The words which are expressed through this relation are called *yogarūḍha* category of words like *paṅkaja* etc.

iv) *Yaugikarūḍhi*

This is the fourth kind of *śakti*. On this category there are various opinions. Some are of the opinion that only three *śāktis* are necessary and the fourth one should not have its existence. But the Naiyāyikas say—no, the fourth type is very much necessary. In this case both etymological and conventional meanings are expressed separately through this *śakti*. Hence the words expressed are called as *yaugikarūḍha* category of words.

Śaktigrahopāya : The means of knowing the relationship between word and meaning.

There are various ways of the apprehension of *śakti* (*śaktigraha*).[13] Some of them are as follows :

(1) *Vyākaraṇa* (Grammar)

Etymology helps in grasping the word meaning relationship. Grammar gives etymology and so it helps in grasping the *śakti*.

(2) *Upamāna* (Analogy)

Analogy helps in grasping *śakti*. For example, when one does not know the meanings of the word *gavaya*, he asks somebody. Then that person says—*go-sadṛśo gavayaḥ*. "A *gavaya* is similar to cow'. Then after seeing the similarity he decides this particular animal is the meaning of the word *gavaya*. This is how anology helps.

(3) *Kośa* (Dictionary)

We know the meaning of words through dictionaries also. Thus a dictionary helps in knowing *śakti*.

(4) *Āptavākya* (Statement of a reliable person)

The statement of a reliable person is sometimes very important to know the meaning of certain words and thereby the relation between the word and its meaning.

(5) *Vyavahāra* (Usage or the observation of verbal communication)

When a child hears an elderly person saying to another person *gām ānaya* 'Bring a cow,' *gām vadhāna* 'tie the cow', *aśvam ānaya* 'bring the horse,' take the pot etc., from such sentences, the child understands the process of bringing, taking, keeping and tying etc. And then he gradually gets acquainted with the meaning of such words as pot, cow, horse, take away, the action of bringing etc. So the learner learns the *śakti* from this observation.

(6) *Vakyaśeṣa* (Verbal description)

In the sentence, '*yavamayaścarūrbhavati*'; here the problem is : what is the meaning of the word *yava* and how to get it ? Whether *yava* refers to 'Barly' or another corn ? But if we look at the description in Vedic literature we find a description.[14] And from that, the meaning becomes clear that the word *yava* here means only 'barly' nothing else. Thus the description helps know the *śakti.*

(7) *Vivṛti* (Paraphrase) :

The meaning is known clearly from the paraphrase of a word or sentence. For example, *ghaṭa* is paraphrased as *kalaśa.* So also the word *pacati* is paraphrased as *pākam karoti* and we come to know that—*ti* means *kṛti.*

(8) *Siddha-pada-sānnidhya* (From the vicinity of a known word)

In the sentence—*iha sahakāratarau madhuram piko rauti.* Here, the word *pika* is understood in the sense of *Kokila* because it is in the vicinity of the word *sahakāra-taru* 'mango-tree'. Hence due to the juxtaposition of a well known word the meaning becomes clear.

These are some of the means to know the relation, but there may be more ways to know the relationship between a word and its meaning.

Notes

1. (i) *Vṛttiśca śābdabodhahetupadārtho-pasthityanukūla padapadārthayoḥ sambandhaḥ. Tat. Ci.* (*Śabda*). p. 627.

(ii) *Vṛttyā padapratipādya eva padārtha ityabhidhīyate Śakti.* p. 5.

2. *Vṛttiśca śaktilakṣaṇānyatara sambandhaḥ Nyā. Si. Muk.* p. 264.

3. *pare tu śābdabodhajanaka padapadārtha sambandhatvam ityāhuḥ.* *Laghumañ* (*Sphoṭavāda*) p. 13.

4. (i) *na sāmayikatvācchabdārtha śampratyayasya. Nyā. Sū* 2.1.55, p. 543.

(ii) *kaḥ punarayam samayaḥ, asya śabdasyedamarthajātamabhidheyamiti abhidhānābhidheya niyamaniyogaḥ Nyā. Bhā.* on *Sū.* 2.1.55, p. 543.

Vārttikakāra and Tātparyaṭikākāra also accept *samaya* in that sense.

5. *kim sambandhamātreṇa, śabdasya hi nijam sāmarthyam śabdatvam. āgantukam ca sāmarthyam saṅketoviśiṣṭā cānupūrvī, tasmādeva sāmarthyadvitayāt tadarthapratyayopapattiḥ, Nyā. Kan.* p. 518.

6. *śaktiśca padena saha padārthasya sambandhaḥ Nyā. Si. Muk.* p. 265.

7. (i) *Sā cāsmācchābdādayamartho bodhavya itiśvarecchārūpaḥ.* Ibid.

(ii) *Idam padamimamartham bodhayatviti asmācchabdādayamartho bodhavya iti vecchāḥ, saṅketarūpā vṛttiḥ Sakti* p. 5.

(iii) *Īvarasaṅketaḥ Śakti*, Ibid.

8. *tatrādhunikasaṅketaḥ paribhāṣā, tayā cārthabodhakam padam pāribhāṣikam pāribhāṣikam yathā sāstrakārādisaṅketita nadī vṛddhyādipadam.* Ibid.

9. *navyāstu īśvarecchā na saktiḥ kintvicchaiva Nyā. Si. Muk.* p. 266.

10. *avayavaśaktiḥ yogaḥ—Tar. Dīp.* p. 51.

11. *samudāyaśaktiḥ rūḍhiḥ*, Ibid.

12. *Yogena sahitā rūḍhiriti*, *Nīlakanṭhī* 4.31.

13. *Śaktigraham vyākaraṇopamāna/kośāptavākyāt vyavahāratașca/vākyasyaśeṣād vivṛter vadanti/sānnidhyataḥ siddhapadasya vṛddhāḥ// Nyā. Si. Muk*. p. 266.

14. *vasante sarvaśasyānām jayate patratāṭanam/modamānāśca tiṣṭhanti yavāḥ kaṇaśasālinaḥ//* Ibid. p. 275.

3.2. *LAKṢAṆĀ*

Lakṣaṇā is called the secondary relation between a word and its meaning. It is conceived by the Nyāya-vaiśeṣika system as a relation with the primary sense of that word.[1] The knowledge of secondary relation depends upon the knowledge of primary relation. In other words *lakṣaṇā* is considered to be a relation when *abhidhā* i.e. the primary sense is not applicable. In such case the primary meaning is obstructed (*bādhita*), then we get *lakṣyārtha* (secondary meaning). Suppose we take an example, that 'man is a lion'. Here the primary meaning is not taken into consideration, but the meaning is accepted figuratively viz. the man has the strength equal to that of the lion.

So when the literal meaning does not fit into the context, there is *mukhyārthabādhā* and then we go for the secondary meaning. To give an example let us discuss the following two sentences :

(1) *Gaṅgāyām ghoṣaḥ* nivasati*

'The milkman lives on the bank of the Ganges.'

(2) *Gaṅgāyām ghoṣaḥ snāti*

'The milkman takes bath in the Ganges.'

In the first case the word *Gaṅga* means—the bank of the Ganges and in the second case the word *Gaṅgā* means—Gaṅgā

---

*In the Bengal tradition, the word *ghoṣaḥ* not only mean *ābhirapalli* but also a milkman.

water. One cannot take the same meaning 'the bank of Ganges' in both the cases. It is because in the case of the example (1) to understand the meaning on the bank of Ganges, one is required to know the primary meaning 'water' of the word *Gaṅgā*. This is the reason that *lakṣaṇā* is defined as *śakya-sambandhaḥ*, 'the relation with the primary meaning.' The reason for going for *lakṣaṇā* is *tātparyānupapatti*,[2] 'inexplicability of the intention of the speaker' and not *anvayānupapatti* 'inexplicability of the relationship with the primary meaning.' For example—in the instance, *yaṣṭiḥ praveśaya*, here the primary meaning of the word *yaṣṭiḥ* is not intended by the speaker when he utters that sentence with an intention that 'the holders of the stick' should be asked to enter in to the dining hall.[3] That is why from the word *yaṣṭi* what is intended is that 'a holder of the stick' and not merely the 'stick'. Thus the ground for resorting to *lakṣaṇā* is *tātparyānupapatti* and not *anvayānupapatti*.

Classification of Lakṣaṇā

Generally *Lakṣaṇā* is divided into three kinds namely—(i) *Jahatśvārthā* (ii) *ajahatsvārthā* and (iii) *jahadajahatsvārthā*. Let us take up individually each one of them and analyse :

(1) *Jahatśvārthā*

This type of *lakṣaṇā* is that where the primary sense is fully abandoned and a new meaning is substituted in its place.[4] The example is given as – *Mañcāḥ krośantī* where the word *mañcāḥ* refers to a child sleeping on an erected seat and not the seat proper. Also in the case of the famous example—*Gaṅgāyām ghoṣaḥ* 'the village is on the Ganges'. This kind of *lakṣaṇā* is sometimes called by the term *jahatsvārtha lakṣaṇā* or briefly *jahallakṣaṇā*. Thus a *jahatsvārthā lakṣaṇā* is that in which the primary meaning of a word is abandoned and replaced by another meaning.

(2) *Ajahatsvārthā*

In this type of *lakṣaṇā*, the word retains its own meaning and conveys something more[5], as in the case of *chatriṇo yānti*. Here in this example—where both those who have umbrellas and those who have not are implied. The other example—*kākebhyo dadhi rakṣatām* where all birds including crows are to be understood from the work *kāka*. The intention is obviously that the curd should be protected not only from crows, but from all other creatures like cats and dogs which are capable of eating the curd.

In the above case, there is no difficulty in accepting *anvaya* and the literal meaning i.e. no obstruction in accepting the primary meaning (*mukhyārtha-bādhā*). But the intention of the speaker was not only to convey the primary meaning of the word *kāka* but *kāketara*, crow as well as other than crow. It is the intention (*tātparya*) of the speaker which decides the real meaning of a sentence when the purpose is not solved merely by the primary or literal sense.

(3) *Jahadajahatsvārthā*

In this type of *lakṣaṇā* only a part of the primary meaning is retained and a part is rejected.[6] For example—*so' yam Devadattaḥ, tattvamasi* etc. In the first example—*saḥ* means 'that Devadatta' (*tatkālīna Devadatta*) and *ayam* means 'this Devadatta'—(*etatkālīna Devadatta*). This conflict is removed when we retain the essential existence (identity) of Devadatta and ignore the differences caused by different factors like time and place etc. In the second example however, the word *tat* refers to *nirguṇa Brahma* and *tvam* denotes *saguṇa jīva*. Hence we leave the properties *nirguṇatva* and *saguṇatva* and make the two substances identical.

Notes

1. *lakṣaṇā śakyasambandhaḥ. Nyā. Si. Muk. Kārikā* 82.
2. *tātparyānupapattiḥ lakṣaṇābījam. Tar. Dīp.* p. 51.
3. *Yaṣṭipraveśe bhojana tātparyānupapattyā yaṣṭidhareṣu lakṣaṇā. Nyā. Si. Muk.* p. 286.

4. (i) *yatra vācyārthasyānvayābhāva-statra jahatī. Tar. Sam*. p. 51.

(ii) *lakṣyatāvacchedakarūpeṇa lakṣyamātrabodhikā jahl-lakṣaṇā. Nyā Bo*. p. 52.

5. (i) *yatra vācyārthasyānvayastratrājahatī yathā chatriṇo gacchanti. Tar. Dīp*. p. 51.

(ii) *lakṣatāvacchedakarūpeṇa lakṣyaśakyobhayabodha-prayojikājahallakṣaṇā. Nyā. Bo*. p. 52.

6. *yatra vācyaikadeśatyāgenaikadeśānvayastatra jahadajahatī yathā tattvamasiti. Tar. Dīp*. p. 51.

4.0. *CONCEPT OF SAMUDĀYA*

In Nyāya system the word *samudāya** stands for 'collection'. The five membered syllogism is a *samudāya* of five sentences.[1] The *Nyāko*[2] mentions that the *samudāya* 'collection' is not different from the individuals or parts (*avayavas*)—*atra smaryate sumudāyaḥ pratyekānatiriktaḥ iti naiyāyikānām siddhānta iti.*

The reality of a collection is not denied. A sentence is a collection of words in a particular order.

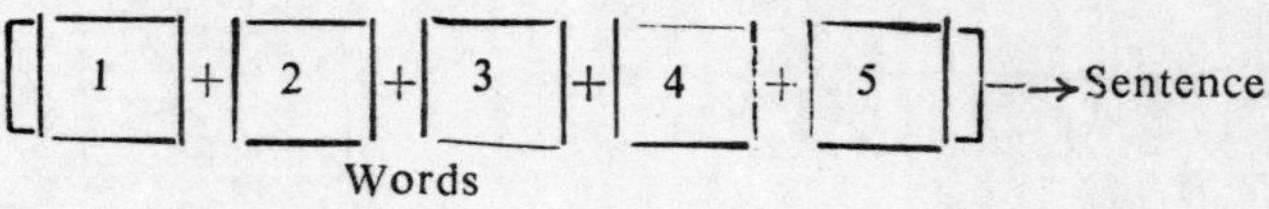

The words first come into existence and then the sentence. Likewise the meanings of the words 'parts' (*avayavas*) are known first, then the meaning of the sentence.

Śāb. Bhā. and *Tan. Vār.* record that the collection is a combination of parts put together i.e. *samudāyasya samudāyibhyaḥ avyatirekaḥ.*[3] That suggests that the collection is not different from the individual parts. This kind of notion of *avayava* and *samudāya* is also described in the *Ślo. Vār.*[4] And when the part is unable to express the desired sense it is expressed through *samudāya.*[5] This is known on the basis of common usage (*loka prasiddhiḥ.*).[6]

In Nyāva philosophy, we find a set of words which express the idea of individuals or constituents and with the help of those constituents a collection is formed. They are—

(1) *samudāya*	*samudāyin*
(2) *sāmagrī*	*samagra*
(3) *saṁhati*	*saṁhanyamāna*

These sets refer to the idea that in a sentence there are various words and by the help of the collection of words we get a sentence. The collection is a sentence. Hence a collection is not a separate entity but merely putting together the words.[7]

But there is also another pair of terms which also express the exact idea with little difference, that is—*avayava* and *avayavī*. Here, the word *avayava* refers to a 'part' and the word *avayavī* refers to a 'whole'. There is a kind of relation existing between the two. One is a cause i.e. *avayava* and the other is the effect *avayavī*. For example, *kapāla* is *avayava* which is a cause of the effect (product) *ghaṭa* (*avayavī*). Both are called entities where as in the earlier sets of words, they are not treated as independent entities. This is the difference maintained between the two sets of terms in Nyāya school. Sometimes we also find that the word *sākalya* is used in the sense of collection.

In the present context the word *samudāya* is to be understood in the sense of collection, or total or whole.

Notes

1. (i) *Pratijñādi—vākyapañcaka-samudāyo nyāyaḥ. Nyā Pra.* p. 95.

   (ii) *Pratijñādy—avayavapañcaka—samudāyatvam. Nyā. Bo.* p. 38.

2. p. 975.

3. (i) *Tan. Vār*, 2.2.5.14.

   (ii) *samudāyasya avayavair-avyatirekaḥ. Śāb. Bhā.* 11. 2. 3. 14.

4. *tasyā-pyatyantabhinnatvam na syād avayavaiḥ saha/ vyaktibhyo jātivac caiva na nikṛṣṭaḥ pratīyate//* *Ślo. Vār.* 18.75.76.
5. *asatsv—avayavārtheṣu yo'nyatrārthe prayujyate/ tatrānanyagatitvena samudāyaḥ prasiddhyati//* *Tan. Vār.* 1.4.8. p. 344.
6. *prātipadikam tāvad—udbhedana samarthe dravye khānitrādāvayavaprasiddhyā pravarttate na ca samudāyo'rthān taravācī loke prasiddhaḥ.* *Tan. Vār.* 1.4.1 p. 322.
7. *Nyā Mañ*, p. 36.

* Notes : In Buddhist philosophy the word is technically used in the sense of the cause of sorrows and sufferings—

samudāyo duḥkhakāraṇam. tad dvividham pratyayopanibandhano hetupanibandhanaśca. Sar. Dar. Sam., p. 40.

4.1. *CONCFPT OF AVAYAVA*

The Mīmāṁsakas and the Naiyāyikas ascribe various meanings to the term *avayava.* One of its meanings is 'a members of syllogism'. In Nyāya system we have the five-membered syllogism i.e. *pañcāvayava vākyam.* Gautama and Vātsyāyana use this term many a time in their texts. In *Nyāya Sūtra* 1.1.32 Gautama enumerates—*pratijñā-hetu-udāharaṇo panaya-nigamanāny—avayavāḥ* That means—*pratijñā, hetu, udāharaṇa, upanaya* and *nigamana* are the five members of syllogism. Vātsyāyana also uses the term in the same sense.[1] In another case he has mentioned that *avayava* means a part of the five membered inference.[2] It can be any part of the five members.

In *Nyāya Bodhinī*[3] it is mentioned as—*pratijñādy-avayava-pañcaka-śamudāyatvam, avayavatvam ca pratijñādy—anyatama-tvam.* When we analyse a sentence meaning, we first understand the meaning of the individual parts i.e. words and its further divided parts and then connecting together, we get the sentence meaning. So words being parts of a sentence are meaningful in themselves. Every word has its own meaning. We know the meanings of these words with the help of etymology. When we want to derive a word, we go to its origins i.e. the grammatical root, the suffix and the like. So these roots and the suffixes are called as *śabdāvayavas.* But the *avayavas* of a word are obtained by the process of derivation and in that respect the science of Grammar helps a lot.

Another meaning is that which refers to a part where there is a whole and part relationship. For example—thread (tantu), is *avayava* 'part' of cloth *paṭa* and 'cloth' is *avayavī* 'whole'. The part is the cause and the whole is the effect produced (product).

The Mīmāṁsakas[4] also have used the term earlier in the above senses which have been followed by the Naiyāyikas.

What is important in the present context is the part and whole relationship.

Notes

1. *sādhanīyasy-ārthasya yāvati śabdasamūhe siddhiḥ parisamāpyate tasya pañcāvayavāḥ pratijñādayaḥ samūham-apekṣāvayavā uchyante. On Nyā Sū.* 1.1.1.
2. *arthasādhaka-bhāvāttu pratijñādayaḥ sādhakavākyasya-bhāgā-ekadeśā vayavā iti. Nvā. Bhā.* on *Sū.* 1.1.32.
3. P. 38.
4. (i) *aśvakarṇā-jakarṇādau samāsā-nugame sati/ apetāvayavārtho' rtho dṛśyate vṛtta śabdavat.// Tan Vār.* 1.3.24. p. 266.

   (ii) *na ca vedāṅga-bhāvo'pi kaścid vyākaraṇam prati/ tādarthyā-vayavā-bhāvāt buddhādi-vacaneṣv-iva.//* Ibid. p. 264.

   (iii) *śruti-liṅgādibhi-stāvattadarthyam nāsya gamyate/ akṛtrimasya vā kaścit-kṛtrimo'vayavaḥ katham//* Ibid. p. 264.

4.2. *SAMUDĀYAŚAKTI*

In Mīmāṁsā system the term *samudāyaprasiddhi* is used instead of *samudāyaśakti* which is found in Nyāya system. There is a *nyāya* that the *samudāyaprasiddhi* obstructs the application of *avayavaprasiddhi*,[1] but not otherwise. They say that when the words like *kuśala* and *pravīṇa* etc. are taken into consideration then etymological meanings will be 'one who cuts kuśa grass' and 'one who plays *vīṇā* nicely'. But in usage *kuśala* means—a skilful person and *pravīṇa* also has the same sense. Here, both these words express the meaning on the basis of *samudāyaprasiddhi*. This *samudāyaprasiddhi* yields *rūḍhyartha*, which is presented to hearer's mind more quickly than the *avayavārtha*. This *nyāya* is called *rūḍhinyāya*.

In Nyāya system the word *samudāyaśakti* is generally used in the sense of conventional relation. It is the expressive relation applied to the whole word which expresses the primary meaning on the basis of usage. This refers to the definition of *rūḍhi* (conventional relation) which is applicable to the whole word. And the word expressive of this kind of relation is called *rūḍha* category of words like—*ghaṭa*, *paṭa*, *go*, *aśva*, *kuśala* etc. Yādavācārya in his *Nyā. Si. Mañ. Sāra* mentions that, the conventional relation is that by which the word expresses the primary meaning through the relation applied to the whole of it.[2] The word which is expressed from time immemorial in a particular sense which is not directly connected with its etymology. Hence the term *rūḍhi* is defined as 'the expressive relation in the whole word without any reference to its parts.[3]

In Mīmāṁsā system, the word is used in the same sense frequently.[4] We also find the usage of *samudāyarūḍhi* in *Tantravārttika.*[5]

Notes

1. (i) *Samudāyaprasiddhir avayavaprasiddher-bādhika-iva samadhigatā. Śāb. Bhā.*, 6.7.22. *p.* 1500.
   (ii) *labdhātmikā hi samudāyaprasiddhir avayavaprasiddhim bādhate. Tan. Vār.*, 1.4.8. p. 344.
   (iii) *samudāyaprasiddhiḥ labdhātmikā avayavaprasiddhim bādhate. na ca samudāyasya apūrvaśaktyantara-kalpanā pramāṇam vidyate. Tan. Vār.*, 2.1-5-17 p. 421.
2. *samasta-śaktigrahaḥ samudāyaśaktigrahaḥ.* p. 181.
3. *samudāyaśaktir-rūḍhiḥ. Tar. Dīp.*, p. 51.
4. (i) *āśvavālaikṣavījaśabdau tu yadi tāvad-vaidika-prayoga-labdha-samudāyaprasiddhitvena laukikīm avayavaprasiddhim jahitas tataḥ siddham eva śāstrastha-pratipatti-balīyastvam. Tan Vār.*, 1.3.9, p. 148.
   (ii) *nirukta-vyākriyādvārā prasiddhiḥ kim valīyasī/ samudāya-prasiddhir-vā mlecchasyaivārtha vā bhavet//* Ibid. 1.3.10, p. 149.
5. *mlecchaprasiddhi vyavahartṛdaurbalye'pi samudāyarūḍhi balena śvarupagatena jyāyasī pratibhāti.* Ibid.

4.3. AVAYAVAŚAKTI

The Nyāya concept of *avayavaśakti* and *samudāyaśakti* is quite similar to the Mīmāṁsakas' concept of *avayavaprasiddhi* and *samudāyaprasiddhi.* Now let us discuss what is this *prasiddhi.* In the *Mīm. Sū.* III. ii. 1-2, Jaimini and his commentator discuss the concept of two varieties of word-meanings namely—*mukhya* and *gauṇa.* While discussing this Śabara mentions that—*prasiddhi*[1] is called *prajñāna* i.e. knowledge of usage. In other words, it is an established fact that such and such words express such and such meaning. Hence the corresponding meanings are called *yaugikārtha* and *rūḍhārtha.* The former is based upon *avayavaprasiddhi* and the latter on *samudāyaprasiddhi.*

The Naiyāyikas use the term *avayavaśakti* in the sense of a relation which expresses the primary meaning of a word. This refers to the definition of *yoga* (etymological relation) which is applicable to the component parts of a word.[2] And the word expressive of this kind of relation is called *yaugika*[3] category of words—like *pācaka* etc. Here the meaning of this word is known from the verbal root *pac*—'to cook' and the suffix-*aka* signifying the agent of the action of cooking.

The word *avayavaprasiddhi* occurs frequently in *Śāb. Bhā.* and *Tan. Vār.* in Mīmāṁsā system.[4] The *avayavaśakti* does not work when there is *samudāya śakti* applicable to a word.[5] That means the *avayavaśakti* is weaker than the *samudāyaśakti* when both are applicable to a word.

Notes

1. (i) *prasiddhiernāma prajñānam.* *Śāb. Bhā.*, 3.2.1-2.
   (ii) *padārtha-pada-sambandha-jñānāpekṣa pravartanāt| prasiddhır-yatra tatrasthā vākyārthāyānugamyate||* *Tan. Vār.* 1.3.5.
2. *avayavaśaktir-yogaḥ.* *Tar. Dīp.* p. 51.
3. *avayava-mātra-śaktikam yaugikam.* *Si. Ca.* p. 88.
4. (i) *prātipadikam tāvad-udbhedana samarthe dravye khanitrādā-vayavaprasiddhyām pravarttate. na ca samudāyo'rthāntara vācī loke prasiddhaḥ......teno' dbhit sādhanako yogo'vagamyate.* *Tan. Vār.*, 1.4.1, p. 322.
   (ii) *avayavaprasiddhyā ājigamanād-ājyāni katham ājigamanam iti arthavādavacanāt.* *Śāb. Bhā.*, 1.4.3. p. 331.
   (iii) *Śāb. Bhā.* 6.7.22, *Tan. Vār.* 1.3.9. p. 223. 1.4.2. p. 327.
5. (i) *labdhātmikā hi samudāyaprasiddhir-avayavaprasiddhim bādhate.* *Tan. Vār.* 1.4.8, p. 344.
   (ii) *samudāyaprasiddhir-avayavaprasiddher-vādhika-iva samadhigatā.* *Śāb. Bhā.* 6.7.22. p. 1500.

5.0. *HISTORY AND DEVELOPMENT OF THE CONCEPT OF YOGARŪḌHI*

The attestation of the word and concept of *yogarūḍhi* goes back to the period of Vāmana. In his *Kā. Sū. Vṛ.* (8th Cent.-9th Cent. A.D.) he mentions that—'*sudatyādayaḥ stry-adhidhāyino yogarūḍha-śabdāḥ*'.[1] He does not say anything more and does not comment on this. He has simply quoted the earlier views. The quotation means that the word *sudatī* is a *yogarūḍha śabda*. But from this, we can say that before his time the word was used and the concept of *yogarūḍhi* was known. We do not get any record about the earlier reference where the word is used and so we do not know who used this term earlier.

Then the famous Naiyāyika Jayanta Bhaṭṭa (Cir. 890 A.D.) uses the term *yogarūḍhi*[2] in a casual manner. In connection with the definition of *pratyakṣa* he refers to the view that some scholars do not accept this category of words. He himself does not accept the *yogarūḍha* category of words. He just records the earlier views of the scholars and does not continue the discussion. So it is clear that before his time, the idea of *yogarūḍhi* was clearly known.

Then comes Sucarita Miśra who wrote a commentary on *Ślo. Vār.* namely *Kāśikā* (1000 A.D.-1100 A.D.). He has used the term frequently in his text and accepts *yogarūḍha* category of words. With reference to the discussion on the word *śāstra*, whether it expresses through *yoga* (etymological relation) or by *rūḍhi* (conventional relation), he says that it expresses through *yogarūḍhi* like the word *paṅkaja*, because in the case of the word *go*, in the expression *gām-ānaya*, even though there is *yoga* '*gacchatī-ti*' but people do not use this in that sense. But it is a *rūḍha śabda* which is conventionally accepted and well-known.

Likewise, the term *śāstra* neither expresses through *yoga* that it instructs us about the attainment of *puruṣārthas* or *śiṣyate anena iti*, nor through *rūḍhi* like *Vedāṅgādi śāstrāṇi*. But it expresses through *yogarūḍhi* 'etymologico-conventional' and hence called a *yogarūḍha śabda*—like the word *paṅkaja*.[3]

Then comes Pārthasārathī Mishra who wrote a commentary on *Ślo. Vār.* namely *Nyāyaratnākara* (1025-75 A.D.), while commenting on the same topic of *śāstra*, he also has discussed in the same manner that the word *śāstra* is neither a *yaugika* word *śiṣyate anena iti*' nor a *rūḍha* word used in the sense of *vedāṅgani śāstrāṇi*. But the word *śāstra* is a *yogarūḍha* category of word like the word *paṅkaja*.[4]

In the text *Sar. Kaṇ.* (1010-1055 A.D.) we find that Bhoja uses the term *yogarūḍhi*. He mentions that *tatra yogarūḍhi-paramparādi-nimittā-padayuktir-yathā*.[5] He quotes the example—*prācyām nirjita jambhajid dvipa śiraḥ sindūra śobham diśi*....and then he says that here the word *jambhajid-dvipa* is a *yogarūḍha*[6] word which refers to the heavenly elephant of Lord Indra i.e. Airāvata. In this context the commentator Ratneśvara in his *Rat Dar.* (14th Cent. A.D.) mentions that the word *jambhajid* is a primary derivative and hence called *yaugika śabda*. But when the same word found in a compound form, namely *jambhajid-dvipa*, it means the elephant Airāvata.[7]

After that we get the direct reference of the term *Yogarūḍha* in the commentary *Ma. Bhā. Pra.*[8] of Kaiyaṭa (11th Cent. A.D.) He clearly states that the word *śabdapārāyaṇa* is a *yogarūḍha* category of words which is used in the etymologico-conventional sense.

Then Śaśadhara in 12th cent. A.D. the author of the text *Nyā. Si. Dī.* introduced this category of words for the first time in Nyāya system. Before him there was nobody who classified words into a detailed manner as he has done in his text. It can be put on record that Śaśadhara the pre-Gaṅgeśa Navya-Naiyāyika has devoted a separete chapter of discussion of the problem of *yogarūḍhi.*[9] He has recorded the earlier views of the opponents. In the beginning he refers to the positions of his opponents that—whether the word *paṅkaja* is expressed through *yoga* i.e. *avayavaśakti* or through *rūḍhi* i.e. *samudāyaśakti* ? References to two groups of opponents have been made. One group is referred to by *eke* and the other by *apare.* Śeśānanta[10] the commentator on *Nyā. Si. Dī.* identifies *eke* as the Grammarians and *apare* as the Bhāṭṭas. The grammarians think that the *avayavaśakti* can itself explain the understanding of lotus arising from the word *paṅkaja,* and the Bhāṭṭas hold that the word *paṅkaja* can be treated as a *rūḍha* word. But Śaśadhara refutes the opponents views and proves that *yogarūḍhi* is necessary for the understanding of the words like *paṅkaja* etc. And hence the corresponding word is called as *yogarūḍha.*

For the first time the definition is supplied by him as—*yaugikārtha-buddhirūpa-sahakāri lābhād—viśiṣtārtho-pasthāpakatvam rūḍheḥ yogarūḍhatvam*—'that *rūḍhi* (word used in conventional sense) is said to be *yogarūḍhi* which presents a qualified meaning to one's mind helped by the knowledge of the etymological sense'.

After Śaśadhara, Gaṅgeśa deals with the problem of *yogarūḍhi* in great detail in his *Śabdakhaṇḍa* of *Tattvacintāmaṇi.* He also raises the opponents view whether *yogarūḍhi* is to be accepted over and above the relations called *yoga* and *rūḍhi.* The opponents do not accept *yogarūḍhi* and say that the primary relations like *yoga* and *rūḍhi* are capable enough to express the meaning lotus from the word *paṅkaja.* But Gaṅgeśa refutes the arguments one by one and establishes his own theory that—*yogarūḍhi* is necessary in such cases. The terms like *paṅkaja, kṛṣṇasarpa* etc. are called *yogarūḍha* category of words. It is observed that Gaṅgeśa follows the same arguments of the opponents recorded by Śaśadhara and develops on those issues and offers his solutions. Finally, he defines *yogarūḍhi* as—*avayava-samudāya-smārita-paṅkajanikartṛ-padmānām paṅkajanikartṛ padmam-ityanubhavo'vayava-samudāyābhyām sambhūya janyate, samudāyopasthita-padmena samam svārthā-nvayo'-vayavair-vā avayavajanitā-nubhavopasthita-paṅkajani-kartṛtvena samam svārthānvayaḥ vā anubhāvyate.*[11] That means the know-ledge of lotus which grows in the mud is produced by both *avayavaśakti* and *samudāyaśakti* together, as lotus which grows in the mud being remembered by *avayava* and *samudāya śakti.* And also the relationship with its meaning is known either by *avayavaśakti* with reference to the lotus which is presented by *samudāyaśakti* or the relationship with its meaning is experie-nced through *samudāyaśakti* with reference to the experience which is presented by that which grows in the mud, which is produced by the *avayavaśakti.*

Cidānanda Paṇḍita in his *Nī. Tat. Bhā.* (12th Cent.-14th Cent, A.D.) has dealt with the problem of *yogarūḍhi* with reference to the word *pratyakṣa.* He accepts that the word *paṅkaja* expresses lotus neither by *yoga* nor by *rūḍhi* but by *yogarūḍhi.*[12]

In *Śa. Śa. Pra*—the words are divided into four categories namely—(i) *yaugika* (ii) *rūḍha* (iii) *yogarūḍha* and (iv) *lakṣaka.* But Jagadīśa mentions that the other variety called—*yaugika-rūḍha* is accepted by others.[13] He argues in favour of *yogarūḍhi* and defines that *yogarūḍhaṁ tu paṅkajādi padam—avayava vṛttyā rūḍhyartham-eva samudāyaśaktyā cā-vayava-labhyārtham-evā-nubhāvayati, na-tv-anyat.* He has also supplied the division of the *yogarūḍha* category of words in to two namely— (i) *sāmāsika*—a compound word like *kṛṣṇasarpa* and (ii) *taddhitānta*—a secondary derivative like *vāsudeva.*[14]

Here *kṛṣṇasarpa* not only etymologically means a black serpent, but through conventional usage—it refers to a parti-cular type of poisonous snake. So also *vāsudeva* can be any son of Vasudeva by the derivation—*vasudevasya apatyam pumān*, but it is restricted to the usage of Lord *Kṛṣṇa* only.

And he remarks that though the word *paṅkaja* is a primary derivative it should be included in the first category called—*sāmāsika.* Thus for the first time such a division of the *yogarū-ḍha* category of words is made in the Nyāya-system.

But Jagadīśa in his *Tarkāmṛta* also mentions the four-fold

classification of words—namely—(i) *yaugika* (*ii*) (*rūḍha* (*iii*) *yogarūḍha* and (*iv*) *yaugikarūḍha.* He says—*śaktam padam caturvidham-yaugikam rūḍham yogarūḍham* and *yaugika-rūḍham.* He also gives the same example of *paṅkaja.*[15]

Coming to grammatical system we find that Nāgeśa Bhaṭṭa in his *Vaiyākaraṇasiddhāntalaghumañjuṣā* deals with the problem while classifying *śakti* in to three categories. He says that the words like *paṅkaja* etc. are called as *yogarūḍha* category of words. He defines *yogarūḍhi* as—*yatra śāstrakalpitā vayavārthānvita viśeṣya-bhūtārtha nirūpitam samudāye bodhakatvam sā yogarūḍhiḥ.*[16] Though he did not include *yaugikarūḍha* under *śakti,* but explains in the same chapter. But he mentions that the word *aśvagandhā* is a *yaugikarūḍha* category of words. The word is expressed conventionally in the sense of an Ayurvedic medicine and etymologically in the sense of a horse-stable.

Besides these above authors there are many more authors after Gaṅgeśa who follow this four-fold classification of the primary relationship between a word and its meaning. Some also divide such words in to three categories only, I have mentioned only a few of them from different systems[17] here. Because more-or-less, the same pattern is followed by all of them and we do not find any innovation.

Notes

1. p. 93.
2. *yogarūḍhistu nāma na sammata-iva viduṣām.* p. 234.
3. *yogarūḍhiriyam paṅkajādivat,* p. 106.
4. *paṅkajādi-vad yogarūḍhy abhyupagamena dharmā-dharmopadeśini caturdasā-ṣṭādaśa vā vidyāsthānāni śāstra-śabdābhīdhānīyakam bhajante-nānyad-iti.* p. 289.
5. p. 258.
6. *atra jambhajid dvipa iti yogarūḍhi-paramparā.* Ibid. P. 258
7. Ibid. P. 258

8. *Vṛhaṣpatir-indrāyeti. Pratipadapāṭhasyā-śakyatvam pratipādayitum-ayam-arthavādaḥ śabdānām iti. śabdapārāyaṇa-śabdo yogarūḍhaḥ śāstra-viśeṣasya.* On *Sū.* 1.1.1.
9. *Yogarūḍhivādaḥ*, p. 54.
10. *Nyā. Si. Dī, Pra. Yogarūḍhivādaḥ.*
11. *Yogarūḍhivādaḥ*, Text No. 163.
12. *atas-tāmarasatva-jāteḥ paṅkaja-śabdavācyam na kevala-yogo, nā'pi kevala-rūḍhiḥ, kintu yogarūḍhi-riti-siddham.* p. 60.
13. *rūḍhañca lakṣakañcaiva yogarūḍhañca yaugikam/ taccaturdhā parai rūḍhayaugikam manyante'dhikam//* verse—No. 16.
14. Verse No. 29.
15. p. 88.
16. p. 89.
17. *Nyā Si. Muk.* p. 315, *Nīlakaṇṭhī*, 4, 31, *Nyā-Pra.* p. 103, *Sid. Ca.* p. 88. *Vyut.* p. 193, *Nyā Mā Vis.* 1-4-10 (5.1.4), *Māme.* 21.5., 20. 7, *Bhā. Kau.* 81-5 (2-1.12), *Bhā Dī.* 1.262.9 (3.3.8), 2.8.8 (3.5.6), *Bhā ci.* 89, 12 (1.1.4), 59.33 (1.1.4). *Vai Bhū.* 149.12 (5.30), *La. Śa*, II 183.12, 261.15, II. 2.4, *Rasa.* 144.12, 144.5, 178.8-9, 189.9, 180.17.

5.1. *ARGUMENTS IN FAVOUR OF YOGARŪḌHI BY THE SYSTEMS OTHER THAN NYĀYA-VAIŚEṢIKA*

Mainly the Bhāṭṭa Mimāṁsakas and the Grammarians were the opponents of the Naiyāyikas in arguments in favour of a third variety of the primary relation. While dealing with the problem of *yogarūḍhi*, Śaśadhara in his *Nyā. Si. Dī.* starts with the opponents views. He mentions that some are of the opinion that *yoga* is enough to express lotus from the word *paṅkaja.*[1] And some others say that *rūḍhi* only can express lotus from the word *paṅkaja*[2]. Śeṣānanta the commentator on *Nyā Si Dī.* in his *prabhā* mentions that *eke* refers to the grammarians and *apare* refers to the Bhāṭṭas. So far the Grammarians earlier to Śaśadhara, are concerned, whatever materials we find available there is no such arguments in favour of *yogarūḍhi.* Bhartṛhari uses the terms like *avayava, samudāya, yoga, rūḍhi, rūḍhayoga* and *śakti.* In his *Vāk.* he has not argued anything in favour of *yogarūḍhi.* It seems that he is not in favour of *Yogarūḍhi.* Only *yoga* and *rūḍhi* are attested in his text.

Among the Bhāṭṭas some do not accept this kind of categorisation of *śakti.* But some accept the *yogarūḍhi* as a separate category of the primary relation over and above the etymology and the conventional relationships. In the *Ślo. Vār.*[3] the problem arises with the word *pratyakṣa.* Whether *savikalpaka* is to be accepted as a *pratyakṣa* because there is a gap between *nirvikalpaka* and *savikalpaka.* The same problem has been thoroughly discussed by Cidānanda Paṇḍita in his *Nī. Tat. Bhā.*, which is a text belonging to the Bhāṭṭa School and written between Cir. 12 Cent. A.D. to 14th Cent. A.D.[4] He has written forty four essays (*vādas*) on the Bhāṭṭa theory of Mīmāṁsā. In the eighth *vāḍa* he has dealt with this problem of *yogarūḍhi* with reference to the word *pratyakṣa.* He starts the argument that how *savikalpaka* is to be treated as meaning *pratyakṣa* ? The *nirvikalpaka* is the first perception (*akṣaja*) and *savikalpaka* is produced by *nirvikalpaka* and hence an indirect product of *akṣa.* So also as *anumāna* can be said to be an indirect result of *akṣa* and as such the word *pratyakṣa* may also stand for *anumiti.*

The Reply is no, it is not acceptable, because the *savikalpaka* type of perception is like the *nirvikalpaka* type which is directly involved by the sense-object contact. The word *akṣaja* is treated just like the word *paṅkaja*, where the similar problem arises.

It is because the conventional relation takes care of the word *paṅkaja.* Well, there is not only *rūḍhi* in case of the word *paṅkaja* because the word is a derivative of *paṅka* and—*ja* (jan) and its components have expressive power. It is not that *rūḍhi* is accepted in order to prevent the use of *saugandhika* 'white water lily' *kumuda* elsewhere. Because elsewhere since there is no usage, the non-usage can be explained *anyatrā-prayogasyā-prayogād-evopapatteḥ*). One cannot argue that *rūḍhi* alone can serve the purpose. Because since the components *paṅka* and *ja* are used individually with their meanings and convey what grows in the mud. Moreover, by accepting *yogarūḍhi,* since the word *saugandhika* is used separately, nobody can stop using the word *paṅkaja* here.

If it is argued that, let there be the postulation of the obstruction of the usage, then on the basis of that obstruction only the problem can be solved, what is the need of accepting *rūḍhi* ?

Here is our answer : In the case of the word *paṅkaja,* there is the primary relation with reference to lotus without keeping aside *rūḍhi.* The *aprayoga* is neither produced nor the obstruction is accepted.[5] The word *paṅkaja* cannot be used in the sense of *padma* without *rūḍhi.* Because, when there is no *avayavaśakti* naturally there will be no *sāmagrī* at all. It is said that by the presence of which something occurs, then that is treated as the *sāmagrī* of that effect. It is also not the case that if there is *śakti* in the part, the whole word must be used. But the word *paṅkaja* is not used in the sense of *Kumuda.* That is why the other variety of the primary relation i.e. *rūḍhi* is postulated.[6]

One can not argue that, the earlier usage is the cause of the later usage, since there is absence of that *prayoga* in the case of the word *paṅkaja* in the sense of 'lily.' Because, if it is so, everywhere the earlier usage will be treated as the cause of later usage and there will be contingency of the absence of *rūḍhi* in the case of the word *aśvakarṇa* and *kṛṣṇasarpa*. Therefore, the ancient usage is not the ground for the usage, but it merely helps knowing the *śakti.*[7]

And since *śakti* is the root cause of the *prayoga*, one accepts *rūḍhi* in the case of the word *aśvakarṇa.* So also in the case of the word *paṅkaja*, the ancient usage is the cause of knowing *śakti.* When *śakti* is known as the root cause of the usage, we also accept *rūḍhi* in the word *paṅkaja*.

One can not argue that since there is conventional relation, the occurence of the meaning lotus becomes possible and hence etymology is not a cause. Because, since elsewhere it works as a cause of the relation and here also it can't be denied in the present context.

It is not the case that, when there is no effect, there will be the state of being a cause. But even though the *sāmāgrī* like the constituents of the word *paṅkaja* are expressive of meanings, it must be accepted that *sāmagri* exists. The components express the meaning whatever grows in the mud. Therefore, it is true that in such cases one cannot stop using the etymological relation which expresses the etymological meaning.[8]

If *rūḍhi* is not accepted then how is the restriction made in the case of lily etc.? To this we say that if only *yoga* is accepted as the cause of the occurence as the relation, then in the case of *kumuda* also the word *paṅkaja* should be used. But it is not the fact. Therefore, how is etymology the only cause ?

To the question that from the restriction of the *avayavaśakti*, the word *paṅkaja* may mean *kumuda*, the answer will be in the same manner that the *sāmagrī* will not operate. And if the ground of restriction is not take ninto consideration, then there will be the absence of any ground for accepting *yogarūḍhi* like the nature of the pre-absence of the usage.

For the acceptance of the third category of the primary relation namely *yogarūḍhi*, if someone asks that, the obstructed primary relation (*pratibandha śakti*) is preferred in order to prevent the meaning and usage of lily from the word *paṅkaja*, our answer is—it is not true, because even though the ground is present in the case of *yogarūḍhi* with reference to lily, there will arise the contingency of the usage because of the absence of the one sided application of *sāmagrī*.

Hence, the *tāmarasatva jāti* i.e. the lotusness as an universal is expressed from the word *paṅkaja*, as lotus which grows in the mud, but neither in the sense of only *yoga* 'etymology' nor in the sense of only *rūḍhi* 'conventional' but established as a case of *yogarūḍhi*[9] the third category of the primary relation.

The word *pratyakṣa* expresses *savikalpaka-jñāna* by *yogarūḍi* and excludes other forms of knowledge which are indirectly produced by the sense-object contact.

Notes

1. *paṅkajādipadānām yoga-eva-ityeke. Nyā. Si. Dī.* p. 54.
2. *rūḍhir ity-apare.* Ibid. P. 54.
3. *nirvikalpakabodhe'pi nākṣam kevalakāraṇam|*
   tatpāramparyajāte vā rūḍhiḥ syāt paṅkajātivat||
   4.130. p. 126.
4. Introduction.

5. *vṛttiḥ paṅkajaśabdasya padme rūḍhinnamuñcataḥ/ aprayoga na cotpādyaḥ pratibandho na cādṛtaḥ//* p. 58.
6. *ato na tanmātram sāmagrīti tadatiriktam śaktyantaram kalpyam.* p. 59.
7. *atha prācīnaprayogasya na prayoga-hetutvam-api tu śaktyavagamakatvam*, Ibid. P. 59.
8. *tad-idam-uchyate-pratītantu yogam na hātum kṣamāmahe iti*, Ibid. P. 59.
9. *atas-tāmarasatva-jāteḥ paṅkajaśabda-vācyatvam na kevala-yogo,nā'pi kevala-rūḍhiḥ, kintu yogarūḍhiriti siddham.* p. 60.

5.2. *ARGUMENTS BY ŚAŚADHARA*

Śaśadhara in 12th Cent. A.D. the author of the *Nyā Si. Dī.* discussed in detail this *yogarūḍha* category of words for the first time in Nyāya Philosophy. He is the pre-Gaṅgeśa Navya-Naiyāyika who has taken up various issues of Navya-Nyāya and wrote twenty-six essays (*vādas*) in his text. While discussing the problem of *Yogarūḍhi* he refers to the views of his opponents. The opponents do not want to accept *yogarūḍha* (etymologico-conventional) as a category of words over and above *yaugika* (etymological) and *rūḍha* (conventional) types of words. The *yaugika* type of words involve *avayavaśakti* (i.e.—the expressive relation in the component parts of a word) and the *rūḍha* category of words involve *samudāyaśakti* (i.e. the expressive relation in the whole word). Since these two relations are capable enough to express the word *paṅkaja* independently why one should accept both for the same word, is the contention of the opponents. Śaśadhara refers to the opponents' view and refutes them one by one by giving sufficient ground. Finally he establishes his own theory i.e. *yogarūḍha* as a distinct category of words. The arguments are just like in a dialogue form and presented nicely. For our present purpose I concentrate on the main grounds on which basis Śaśadhara argues in favour of *yogarūḍhi.*

(1) *Opponents*

The main objection raised is why we should postulate *samudāyaśakti* in the word *paṅkaja* ? They give the ground that (i) should it be accepted for the understanding of the meaning lotus-ness or (ii) should it be accepted for excluding the understanding of lily etc. from the word *paṅkaja*[1] ? They hold that the Ist alternative is not tenable, because even without accepting *samudāyaśakti* there can be verbal understanding from the expression *paṅkaja.* This is possible through *saṁskāra* (impression) as in the case of the word *ākāśā* 'sky' in the sentence *ākāśam dravyam.*

Reply :

The *siddhāntin's* reply to opponents (1) from the word *paṅkaja* due to *saṁskāra*, if one regularly gets the knowledge of *padmatva*, then even a person who does not understand the language will have the knowledge of lotus from the sentence *paṅkajam ānaya* which is absurd. So what would be the regulating factor here ?

Obviously, it is the relationship between a word and its meaning which can regulate the situation. In other words, the person who has the knowledge of the relation of the word *paṅkaja* as a whole with lotus alone, can have the verbal understanding of lotus and not any other person.[2]

With reference to the counter example of the understanding of *ākāśatva* from the word *ākāśa* by *saṁskāra* we can say that it is not always true that one invariably remembers *ākāśa* as the material cause of sound. Only occasionally, it is remembered like that and hence we do not allow the permanent relationship of the word *ākāśa* with *ākāśatva.* So, on the other hand, in the case of the word *paṅkaja* however, one who knows the language i.e. one who knows the relationship between *paṅkaja* and its referent, alone invariably understands the lotusness from it. So *saṁskāra* cannot be the regulating factor.[3]

In connection with the second alternative doubt, we can simply state that, such a doubt has no ground. Because the word *paṅkaja* has no primary relationship with *kumuda* and hence *kumuda* cannot be remembered from word *paṅkaja.* And when it is not remembered where is the chance of its being excluded ? No one postulates *śakti* in a word like *ghaṭa* etc. in order to exclude the remembrance of cloth etc.

(2) *Opponents*

It should not be agrued that we need *samudāyaśakti* in order to remember *padmatva* which will debar the use of the word *paṅkaja* for *kumuda*. Because the *avayavaśakti* itself will take care of it.

Reply :

This above argument is not tenable because, it is experienced that a person who does not know the language still he is found to move to bring lily, frog and moss etc. after hearing the word *paṅkaja*.[4] This implies that unless we restrict the relationship by *samudāyaśakti* it is not possible to regularly convey lotus from the word *paṅkaja*.

(3) *Opponents*

They further point out that if one treats the word *paṅkaja* as common words, there will be no problem. Because a particular understanding can take place due to the particular intention of the speaker. So even if the word *paṅkaja* may apply to various etymological senses, what is intended by the speaker can be known from the context. Hence there is no need of *samudāyaśakti*.

Reply :

Śaśadhara replies to the above argument and says—it is not acceptable. Because does the word *paṅkaja* cause the verbal understanding of a particular lotus ? Or does it cause the understanding in which that particular appears as the qualifier[5] ?

The first alternative is not true. Because *padmatva* will not appear in the cognition from the word *paṅkaja*. Similarly, the second alternative is also not acceptable, because it is not yet decided whether in that qualifier there is primary relationship or not. If one accepts primary relationship, then one will have to take resort to *lakṣaṇā*[6] which is not admissible because one experiences the verbal understanding from the word *paṅkaja* in which the referent of the word *paṅkaja* appears as the primary sense.

(4) *Opponents*

After so much discussion still the opponents are not prepared to accept *samudāyaśakti*. They say that well, if you accept *samudāyaśakti* in the word *paṅkaja*, then you will have to take resort to *lakṣaṇā* in the sentence *paṅkajam kumudam ānaya*. Since here the word *paṅkaja* is a qualification of *kumuda* and therefore, it is used in etymological sense only.

Reply :

Śaśadhara refutes this objection and replies—your doubt has no foundation. Because as you are aware that there are several factors involved as the cause of a verbal understanding. One such factor is compatibility (*yogyatā*). So if some meaning is found to be incompatible it will automatically be set aside and in its place a compatible meaning will be supplied. So naturally in the case of the sentence—*paṅkajam kumudam ānaya* also let us maintain that there is *samudāyaśakti* in the word *paṅkaja* and hence *padmatva* will be remembered from it.[7] Still its relation with *kumuda* is incompatible, the *avayavaśakti* alone will function and will supply the etymological sense to be related with lily.

(5) *Opponents*

If the intention of the speaker is treated as one of the causes of verbal understanding, then even a perceived object can be related to the word-meaning. For instance, if some one asks : *kiṁ pacati* ? And if the listener is seen cooking *kalāya* and if he simply intends to convey *kalāya* without uttering the word *kalāya* even the *kalāya* will form the object of the verbal understanding.

Reply :

The *siddhāntin* says that since we do not hold the view that the intention of the speaker is the cause of verbal understanding, we can't accept your suggestion. The function of the intention of the speaker is only to help remember the meaning of a particular word in the case of *lakṣaṇā* and it does not cause the verbal understanding.

(6) *Opponents*

Along with the main argument one issue came up for discussion and it was whether we should accept *arthādhyāhāra* or *śabdādhyāhāra*. The opponents hold the view that the *arthādhyāhāra* alone is proper, because it is logically simpler.

Reply :

It is not acceptable. Because if it is a case of verbal understanding the contents of it must come from the words which are arranged in a particular sequence. Thus, *śabdādhyāhāra* alone will be a proper method.

(7) *Opponents*

The next question raised by the opponent is that what type of meaning is remembered from the word *paṅkaja* which forms the content part of the verbal understanding.

Reply :

Śaśadhara replies : there is no problem. The meaning which is remembered from the word *paṅkaja* in the sentence *paṅkajaṁ ānaya* is 'the lotus which grows in the mud'. The *avayavaśakti* will supply the meaning part 'that which grows in the mud' and the *samudāyaśakti* will identify it as lotus.[8] Thus there will be no difficulty in getting the final meaning 'the lotus which grows in the mud'.

(8) *Opponents*

Further they ask why there is no *yogarūḍhi* in the word *go* which is derived from the root *gam*+the suffix—*ḍo* (o).

Reply :

Our answer is very clear. The etymology of the word *go* as the root *gam*+the suffix—*ḍo* does not seem to be natural one. But somehow the etymology of the word *go* is given with the help of the *uṇādi* rule *gamer ḍoḥ*. Therefore, we do not accept the word *go* as *yogarūḍha*.

(9) *Opponents*

Well, in that case as the word *go* is not *yogarūḍha*, so also the words like *dhenu* etc. should not be derived from root *dhe*+ suffix *nu*.

Reply :

It is uot proper to hold such view. Because there are many such words like *jānu* 'knee', *dānu* 'prosperity' and *bhānu* 'sun' etc. which exhibit the suffix—*nu* and hence it becomes necessary to accept the etymology of the words like *dhenu* etc. as root *dhe*+*nu* etc.

Thus, it has been sufficiently demonstrated why one requires *samudāyaśakti*. Now lastly, Śaśadhara wants to give his own definition of the term—*yogarūḍhi* as—*yaugikārtha-buddhirūpa-sahakārı-lābhād-viśiṣṭārthopasthāpakatvam rūḍheḥ yogarūḍhatvam* : that *rūḍhi* is said to be *yogarūḍhi* which presents a qualified meaning to one's mind helped by the knowledge of the etymological sense.

Notes

1. *kimartham samudāyaśaktikalpanam. padmatva-pratītyartham vā kumudādi apratītyartham vā. Nyā Si Dī.* p. 54.
2. *dṛśyate cātra vyutpattigrahāpekṣā. Kathamanyathā pratyekam vyutpannasya puṁsaḥ paṅkajam-ānayeti śrutavato' pi na padmānayanānubhavo yathā samudāye vyutpannasya.* Ibid p. 56.
3. *tatra hi kadācid aṣṭadravyabhinnatvam kadācit śabdasamavāyitvam, saṁskāravaśād bhāṣate, atra tu vyutpannasya padmatvam niyamena bhāṣate iti mahān viśeṣaḥ.* Ibid, p. 57.
4. *ataeva avyutpannaḥ paṅkajam-ānayeti vākyaśravaṇāntaram kumudādyānayane dolāyate.* Ibid. P. 57.
5. *vastugatyā yo viśeṣaḥ tadbobhakatvam vā viśeṣa prakāreṇa vā.* Ibid. P. 57.

6. *netaraḥ lakṣaṇāpātāt*. Ibid. P. 57.
7. *na ca paṅkajam kumudam ānaya ityatra paṅkajapade lakṣaṇā. Kintu padmatvam upasthitam-api anvayā-yogyatayā nānveti. avayavārtha eva paramanveti iti na kiñcid anupapannam*. Ibid. P. 57.
8. *tatra paṅkajapadena pratyeka-samudāyaśakti-pratisandhāna sahakāri vaśāt-milita-gocaram ekam-eva smaraṇam janyate*. Ibid p. 59.

5.3. *ARGUMENTS BY GANGEŚA*

At the outset Gaṅgeśa presents all the arguments made by the opponents for not accepting the category of words called *yogarūḍha.* The opponents argue that let the word *paṅkaja* stand for lotus with the help of *rūḍhi* and hence it can come under *rūḍha* category of words. Gaṅgeśa takes up all those arguments one after the other and comments on those opponents views and establishes his own view finally. The main arguments are illustrated here.

The opponents pose the question whether the term *paṅkaja* stands for lotus which is the expressed sense of that word ? It is because the *avayavaśakti* is not capable of expressing lotus from the word *paṅkaja* which stands for the primary meaning 'the lotus which grows in the mud'. The understanding of lotus from the word *paṅkaja* is possible through *rūḍhi* 'the conventional relation' i.e. by the help of *samudāyaśakti.*

The contingency is raised by the author that if *rūḍhi* is accepted then there will arise the contingency of the knowledge of the usage of the word *paṅkaja* in the sense of lily (*kumuda*).

Objection

Well, when *rūḍhi* the conventional relation is accepted to express lotus from the word *paṅkaja*, why should not there be both the usage and the knowledge from the primary relation ? The answer is this : it cannot be, because the conventional meaning obstructs the occurence of the primary relationship. This is the view of the old school.

Reply :

We however reply to the above argument that through convention we remember the meaning lotus only through the suffix—*ḍa* which expresses an individual by the rule *janer ḍoḥ*. We experience it in the form of that which grows in the mud which is substantiated by a rule that the linguistic elements expressive of individuals express a particular individual adjacent to it. They supply one example in—*Āgneyi* which ends in *ḍhak* suffix, what is understood is a particular *ṛk* (*mantra*) expressed by the *ḍhak* which is adjacent to it on the basis of context etc.

So in each and every case there exist the factors which cause the experience of lotus only and hence there is no ground to understand lily nor the usage from the word *paṅkaja*.

Objection :

Well, in such case let there be only the conventional relation *rūḍhi*, because we can get both the knowledge and the usage. Then what is the necessity of accepting a third type of relationship called *yogarūḍhi* i.e. which incorporated both the etymological as well as conventional meanings ?

Reply :

No, your proposal is not tenable because the primary relationship (*yoga*) is already established by the help of *avayavaśakti* and also the primary meaning *yaugikārtha*) is experienced. The knowledge of the experience itself is the distinguishing factor in such case if somebody experiences either the etymological meaning or the conventional meaning.

Objection :

Here the Mīmāṁsakas argue that there is no necessity of accepting *śakti* for the remembrance of the meaning 'lotus'. Because the remembrance of meaning is possible on the basis of *saṁskāra* 'impressions'. This impressions take place in the case of the usage of the word *paṅkaja* by the help of the invariable experience of 'lotus'. According to the Mīmāṁsakas, there is a rule that a remembrance is always caused by an impression. They have the objection that—the expressive power of a word *śakti* is not required for experiencing that meaning lotus because the experience that 'the lotus which grows in the mud' is possibly obtained from the parts of the word *paṅkaja*, by the help of the rule that the suffix *ḍa* expresses the individual linguistic elements adjacent to the root.

To the above proposal if someone asks that how then the word *paṅkaja* stands for lotus without *śakti* being involved ?

Opponents' Reply :

We have the following to say :—

The individual elements of the word *paṅkaja* produce the knowledge of lotus with reference to the suffix—*ṅa* depending upon the earlier usage.

Objection :

The opponents doubt is being raised—for regular remembrance there should be impression being regularly stimulated. Since there is no regular stimulator other than *śakti*, there won't arise regular remembrance.

Reply :

It is not the case, because sometimes we normally observe that, even though *śakti* is present, the impressions are not stimulated and hence there is no remembrance of the meaning. And sometimes even without *śakti* the remembrance of *śakti* occurs. And also there is no fixed stimulator because sometimes it breaks the law of concomitance through the knowledges of similarity, the expressive power of a word and the relatum.

But when there is remembrance, a stimulator which arises at that time is postulated which is not an uniform stimulator. This is fixed on the basis of the effect because the properties which are to be postulated are postulated as per the effect.

Objection :

The objections of the Naiyāyikas are raised as follows :—

One argues that there will be contingency of remembrance of the pervader of lotusness of the usage of the word *paṅkaja* in the sense of *kumudatva* 'lilyness' etc.

Reply :

The opponents reply that it is not proper because a stimulator is postulated on the basis of the remembrance and if there is remembrance, there will be no postulation of any stimulator. Therefore, without *śakti,* lotusness is regularly remembered as *śakti* is remembered without *śakti.*

Objection :

If somebody says that there is no necessity of accepting *śakti* in the words like *go* 'cow' etc., because on the basis of the impression at the time of the the usage of the word *go*, the remembrance of the meaning 'cow' is possible, then ?

Reply :

No, it is not so that one accepts *śakti* for the remembrance of the meaning 'cow' etc. But it is true that *śakti* is accepted for causing the experience, because from any source other than the word 'cow' the experience of the meaning 'cow' is not possible. And also a person who does not know the relationship between a word *go* and its meaning 'cow', does not get the verbal understanding of '*cow*'. And also because through *avayavaśakti* (of the constituents of the word *paṅkaja*) we get the knowledge of 'lotus' and hence *samudāyaśakti* is not the cause of that knowledge. That is why it is not proper to postulate *samudāyaśakti* on the basis of experience.

Objection :

Well, let the word *go* be expressive of the contentness. And the remembrance of the meaning 'cow' occurs through impression, if it is so then—

Reply :

It is not proper, because it is necessary to postulate *śakti* with the knowledge of 'cow' which will explain the usage of the word *go*, but not the knowledge of the content, as the content does not explain such usage. And also it is true that nobody will have the experience of the content of the knowledge from the word *go*.

Objection :

Well, if somebody argues that in the sentence *gaṅgāyām ghoṣaḥ*, the remembrance of 'bank' is possible through impressions then there will arise the contingency of not accepting such category of words having secondary relation. And one need not postulate *lakṣaṇā* for the experience of the 'bank', because that experience is possible by the help of other word of that sentence. So regularly remembrance is caused by the relationship between a word and its meaning (*vṛtti*). And hence from the word *paṅkaja* regular remembrance of lotus occurs on the basis of *śakti* as the relationship and because there is no *lakṣaṇā* involved. If it is so—then?

Reply :

It is not true, because in the sentence like *Gaṅgāyām ghoṣaḥ* without a *vṛtti* the meaning 'bank' etc. are not possible and as a result the meaning of the case—endings cannot be related to it. Because there is a rule that the case—suffixes generate the understanding of its own meaning when connected with the meaning of the word. The lotus, however, is conveyed by the phrase—*paṅkaja* and it is possible to relate the meaning of the case ending after the word meaning is remembered like the word *pācaka* 'one who cooks'.

Objection :

In a verbal understanding the relation of one word-meaning is connected with another word-meaning. If this is not accepted, then the meaning of *pacati* will get related to *kalāya* when perce ived by eyes.

Reply :

It is not the case because the speaker does not intend so. An d if he intends then it is possible when someone asks—what are you cooking, and the daughter in-law shows *kalāya*. In that case *kalāya* will form the content of the verbal understanding. Otherwise why is it not that, such a relation is possible from the word *kalāya* either heard or remembered by chance?

Objection :

Another objection is raised in this connection that the *śabdādhyāhāra* is not important but *arthādhyāhāra* is enough for verbal understanding. In the case of the expression *dvāram* one does not supply the word *pidhehi*, but he supplies only the meaning 'close', since it is logically simpler to get the complete sense of that sentence.

Reply :

One need not argue that *arthādhyāhāra* is the cause of verbal understanding. Because in the sentence *padmam ānaya* the understanding of lotus is caused by the word *padma* and elsewhere also the same rule should be applied. For the understanding of lotus, the word *padma* is the necessary cause as having the intention of the speaker for the understanding of lotus related with the action of bringing but not simply word, because it is a cumbersome process. Hence, *śabdādhyāhāra* should be accepted. Because, after one word is uttered the respective meaning is remembered and not directly.

Objection :

Let the word *paṅkaja* be used for lotus when it is coming up in mud at a particular moment and should not be used when that time of growing is over. Because the word *daṇṇī* is used when the man is having a staff.

Reply :

It is not acceptable, because as in the word *pācaka* the suffix expresses the meaning as possessing the action of cooking, so also in the word *paṅkaja* the suffix is capable of referring to the state of lotus even after the time of its birth. Otherwise, even in the case of *yogarūṇhi* one should use the word *paṅkaja* only at the time of its being born.

Objection :

The opponents argue that even that the neo-logicians hold the view that, when there is incompatibility, with the remembered meaning *padma* 'lotus', there arises the knowledge of *kumuda* 'lily' and one does not call it *lakṣaṇā*. But as a matter of fact, when *padmatva* has no capacity to relate itself 'lily' is understood only through primary relation but not through *lakṣaṇā*.

Reply :

It is true that, a person who knows the language regularly remembers the meaning which is the counter-relatum of the relation after he grasps the word and hence the knowledge of the word should be treated as the manifester of impression which is seen in each case and also it is logically simpler. But one need not postulate endless number of unseen factors arising at that time of the remembrance of meaning of that word because it is cumbersome. Therefore, for the remembrance of the meaning *padma*—the knowledge of the word *paṅkaja* should be considered as the manifester of impression and thereby the primary relationship is established.

Objection :

The opponents hold that the word *rathakāra* is not to be accepted for a particular caste conventionally because it is possible to remember that when the impression is manifested.

Reply :

This will lead to a contradiction of the Mīmāṁsā view—that in the sentence 'in the rainy season the *rathakāra* should perform *agnyādhāna* sacrifice, since it is the conventional meaning which is stronger than the etymological meaning, the particular caste will be presented to the mind quicker and hence it suggests that the *ādhāna* rite is enjoined for that particular caste only.

Objection :

They further say that, let one remember lotus from the

word *paṅkaja* since there is a relation of the form of regular usage of the word *paṅkaja*. Hence the relation of the suffix meaning with lotus and its appearance in the verbal understanding become explicable because the understanding is caused by the word *paṅkaja*.

Reply :

It is not proper to say that, the relation of the suffix meaning with lotus and the appearance of the relation in the verbal understanding are helped by the relation between word and its meaning because in the sentence *pācakam ānaya* there is no *vṛtti* present with reference to that which is presented to our mind by that sentence.

Objection :

The opponents raise the doubt that the remembrance of the word-meaning is caused by the *padavṛtti* alone.

Reply :

It is not true that the remembrance is caused by *padavṛtti* but from the knowledge of the relata a *vṛtti* help the remembrance of a meaning as a relation. Otherwise, from a word one cannot remember the primary relation. The primary relation is accepted for verbal understanding of the relations of word meanings. So without *vṛtti* the knowledge of lotus from the word *paṅkaja* is not possible. And hence there is no need of taking resort to the secondary relation in this connection.

Objection :

The opponents say that the word *paṅkaja* can be treated as indicator of lotus but not as expressive of *padma*. They also provide an inference that the word *paṅkaja* is expressive of the meaning lotus, because it regularly causes the remembrance of lotus as in the case of the word *padma*. It is also not tenable.

Reply :

We have the following to answer : As there arises the regular remembrance of *padma* from the word *paṅkaja* by the help of *vyāpti* there will arise the contingency of remembering that which is pervaded by and pervader of *padma*. Since there is only usage in *padma* and usage of *padma* only of the word *paṅkaja* by such constant relation, let there be the remembrance of *padma* alone.

Objection :

They hold that the primary relation is established by the regular usage, because it is not attained by any other way.

Reply :

It is not true, because in such case, the knowledge of the usage will be the probans to establish the probandum. Then one who has seen the usage in a few cases he will not have the knowledge of *vyāpti* and there won't arise the regular remembrance of *padma*. And also the very usage will cause the inferential cognition, and there will arise the contingency that one who has no knowledge of the usage will also have the regular remembrance of lotus.

Objection :

The opponents suggest that with the help of *tarka* the knowledge of *śakti* is generated and then let that knowledge of *śakti* be the cause of the remembrance of the meaning *padma* assisted by *tarka*.

Reply :

If it is accepted then even from the word *go* 'cow' etc. there will arise the remembrance and verbal understanding of cow from the knowledge of the intended usage which causes the knowledge of the *śakti*.

Objection :

The opponents have the following doubt in their mind- whether the regular remembrance of a meaning is possible on the basis of *śakti* or on the basis of regular relation or on the basis of *vṛtti* ? From these the answer is—on the basis of *śakti* the remembrance is possible. They also further say that the *śakti* is remembered and with reference to that there is no difficulty.

Reply :

It is not correct *Śakti* is a relation and it is not remembered but the word meaning is remembered. Because if we accept that then it will involve a cumbersome process and also because without the remembrance of the relata, the remembrance of the relation is not possible. Therefore, it is necessary to remember the word meaning first. To the argument that *śakti* forms a part of the content of the remembrance of the meaning because of the manifestation of the impression. Our reply is it is not proper, because the word is capable of reminding its meaning when uttered but not merely being associated with *śakti.*

Objection :

To the argument that whether the regular remembrance is based on the knowledge of a regular relation only ?

Reply :

The answer is that by the help of *śakti* the word is regularly related as being the locus of that *śakti.* As *śakti* does not require to be known by another knowledge of *śakti* when it is used as a relation. Still *śakti* is known by its nature. It is not a necessary factor for generating the verbal understanding but it is presented as the delimitor of the state of being a producer of the experience. It amounts to the view that *śakti* appears to be a relation when the knowledge of the word meaning is produced.

Objection :

The Mīmāṁsakas argue that let the conventional sense *rūḍhi* obstruct the etymological sense i.e. *yoga* for remembering 'lily'.

Reply :

No, it is not proper, because one can not say that the regular remembrance of lotus is the only obstructing factor for the occurence of 'lily', because there will be no regular remembrance without *rūdhi.* And that is why the rule regarding the suffixes capable of expressing an individual is not accepted.

And also a particular word is used in one sense only and so there is no chance of arising another knowledge of the meaning of the word *paṅkaja.* That means, at the time of one utterance it will stand for a particular sense with the *śakti* being the helping factor as a relation. And also because of the difference maintained in both *avayavaśakti* and *samudāyaśakti.*

Objection :

To the main objection of the opponents if it is said that the *samudāyaśakti* obstructs the *avayavaśakti*—then ?

Reply :

The answer is given as follows : It is not true because in the case of the word *lambakarṇa* there is no obstruction with reference to the action of bringing conveyed through primary relation and also because many meanings are experienced in the case of the polysemous word. And that is why one should not say that one *śakti* obstructs the other.

Objection :

Another doubt is raised to the above issue. They argue that while the remembrance of the *avayavaśakti* takes place then invariably there will be remembrance of *samudāyaśakti.* And hence one remembrance will obstruct the other.

Reply :

The answer is given that it is not true, because whole is identical with parts and so from that whole the remembrance of both the relations are possible. The example like the word *maṇḍapa* can be taken into consideration here. Here both the meanings are equally possible : (i) one who drinks gruel (through *avayavaśakti*) and (ii) a pandel—(through *samudāyaśakti*). But in such case of the word *maṇḍapa* etc. *śakti* is established as being the generator of experience. And hence there is no obstruction of one *śakti* over the other.

But Gangeśa says that the word *śakti* is technical with reference to the obstructor in general. But if *śakti* is established as the causer of the understanding, there will be mutual dependency and if it is understood as an obstructor *śakti* is not established.

Objection :

The opponents argue that whether from the nature of the word *pankaja* and by the help of *ḍa* (a) suffixes from the word *pankajani*, there does not arise the knowledge of 'lily'.

Reply :

Indeed, there does not arise the common experience of *kumuda* etc. from the word *pankaja*. In that case—they may have the following doubts in their mind.

(i) Is it that a person who knows the etymological sense does not get knowledge from that word ? or (ii) Is it that lotus is experienced as that which grows in the mud ?

To these questions we have the following answer : To the first alternative we say that how is it that from the word *pankaja* an experience does not arise when all factors are present as it is in the case of the word *manduraja* 'one who is born in a stable' ?

To the second alternative we remark that *kumuda* should also be remembered because we do not see any difference in the meaning 'that which grows in the mud'.

Objection :

The opponents further argue that, since the word *pankaja* is a common term, by the help of the intention of the speaker the knowledge of lotus and lily are possible. Therefore, it is not necessary to go for conventional or secondary relation at all.

Reply :

The above argument is not proper. Because if one accepts that *padma* and *kumuda* are treated as equal then one who has not known the usage of *pankaja* being used for lily, there will not arise the knowledge of *kumuda*, because of the impossibility of relation with *padma*. And also when one does not know the usage of lily for *pankaja* since there is no relation with lily, there will not arise the knowledge of *padma*. This is the ground for which we accept *rūḍhi* in *padma*. And for *kumuda* we have a separate relation called *lakṣaṇā* and there is no difficulty of understanding lily from the word *pankaja* with the secondary relation.

Objection :

To the doubt that through *rūḍhi* there arises both the usage and the knowledge of *kumuda* from the word *pankaja*. The Naiyāyikas have the following to answer.

Reply :

It is not true, because from the components *paṅka* etc. one experiences lotus only and since we have postulated the restriction in the *avayavaśakti* there does not arise the usage and the knowledge of *kumuda*.

The Naiyāyikas also ruled out the possibility of the opponents view regarding the acceptance of *rūḍhi* in case of *pankaja* that even though there is etymology in the case of the word *pankaja* there is no usage of that word in the sense of *kumuda* where as in the case of the word *udbhid* both the meanings are possible. On the basis of etymology the word is used in the sense of spade and on the basis of conventional sense it is used in the sense of a particular rite. Thus the possibility of only *rūḍhi* with reference to the word *pankaja* is ruled out.

Objection :

To the question that in the word *udbhid*, the primary meaning is not proper to be related to a particular rite, since the etymological sense is obstructed by the conventional sense.

Reply :

It is not true, because when the etymological sense is related to spade, it is due to the primary relation, that the word *udbhid* is used.

Objection :

The *Mīmāṁsakas* argue that it is observed that in the case of the person who knows the relationship of the usage of the word *pankaja* to lotus, the usage cause the knowledge of lotus only and so let us postulate that, it is the nature of the word *pankaja* which conveys lotus. Because the very nature itself, the knowledge of the usage like the knowledge of the relationship is possible to be the auxiliary factor.

Reply :

It is not tenable because it is not good to postulate that the nature of words causes the understanding of meaning but it surely depends upon the knowledge of the relationship. It is because when one does not know the relationship, no understanding is possible from a word. Even for a false knowledge, illusory knowledge of relation is necessary. It is again substantiated that when there is no expressive relation, there won't be any understanding as per the logic when there is no effect suggests that there is no cause.

Objection :

Due to the nearness of the use of the prefixes, as the root meaning gets changed to convey the knowledge of excelling etc. and since there is no auxiliary factor, the understanding of *kumuda* does take place.

Reply :

It is not proper, because the roots with the auxiliary factors of nearness of the prefixes express excellence not merely by itself but through the primary relationship.

Objection :

The arguments regarding the restriction of *avayavaśakti* and the usage of *kumuda* from the word *pankaja* are considered here. The opponents argue that in the pronoun *aham* 'I' etc. the state of being in the mind, being the object of address and being the speaker are the prompting factors of usage and hence that word *aham* refers to that person who is in the mind but that being in the mind is not the expressed sense of the pronoun *aham*. Because, from that pronoun *aham* the knowledge of those factors does not arise. Likewise let lotusness be treated as a prompting factor.

Reply :

It is not tenable. Because, by that the *avayavaśakti* is not restricted as the word *paṅkaja* refers to lotus through the etymological sense also. The intention to lily also is not ruled out because without the obstructing factor the understanding occurs. The *avayavaśakti* is not contradicted because when the factors like expectancy, proximity etc., *śakti* and the intention the speaker are present, naturally there arises the verbal understanding and hence these are not the extraneous factor which is not the cause of the obstructing factor of the verbal understanding.

And also nobody can obstruct the usage, because if the grounds of usage are present namely—the knowledge of *iṣṭasādhanatā* to know the desired lily, on the knowledge of being the volition inferred on that ground, the non-usage cannot be the ground.

Coming to the words like *aham* the self only is the expressed meaning and considering the knowledge of the relation as the auxiliary cause by its very nature only *uccārayitṛtva* 'the state of being an utterer regulates the verbal understanding. And also because of the very nature of the word, that causes the knowledge of 'self' and hence by itself '*uccārayitṛtva*' is called as *upādhi*.

As a matter of fact, this is not the case with lotus-ness, because the common experience of *kumuda* and lotus is an experienced fact.

Objection :

The opponents argue that since *pankaja* is not used earlier in the sense of *kumuda* so there is no later usage in that senses.

Reply :

It is not the case, because one need not ask for the ground for an usage in general.

Objection :

Again the opponents have the following in their mind—The usage is not caused by a group of usage, but it occurs individually. The earlier usage is the ground for the later usage like the earlier usage of the word *go* for the later usage.

Reply :

It is not proper, because the earlier usage is not the ground for later usage because even without the knowledge of the earlier usage, there arises the verbal understanding for one who knows the *avayavaśakti* in words like *pācaka* etc. and the new literary compositions. There arises the perfect usage without any difficulty.

Objection :

The opponents further ask that in the case of the word *grāmagāma*, since there is no understanding, the knowledge of correctness also should be considered as the ground.

Reply :

One cannot argue that the knowledge of correctness be the ground for understanding. The important factor is the necessity of accepting *śakti* and let the knowledge of distinction between *gauṇa* and *lākṣaṇika* be maintained on the basis some *upādhi* and absence of some *upādhi*. Because the knowledge of the word becomes the cause by the first usage and hence in that word one postulates *śakti*. But in the word *grāmagāma* there is logical difficulty like the expectancy etc. and hence one postulates the knowledge of correctness as the cause.

Objection :

The opponents define correctness '*sādhutva*' as that which is not the continuation of the earlier usage since it is absent in new literary compositions, but it is the absence of being produced by illusion of relationship. In the case of the usage *kumuda* also because of the illusion of that relationship, the usage of the word *pankaja* is usually found.

Reply :

It is not proper that since there is the state of being produced by illusion, there is the state of not causing understanding and since it is causing understanding there is the state of being produced by illusion. As a result it leads to the fault of mutual dependency. Because the state of being produced by earlier illusion becomes the cause of the later illusion and hence the later usage is an illusion. And like that it leads to a chain of illusions which is a fact also in the word *grāmagāma.*

And if asked how this illusion is known ? The answer is as the word *grāmagāma* is understood so also an authoritative person does not use the word *pankaja* for *kumuda* without any extraneous factor.

Objection :

The opponents argue that by the help of illusion of the factor of correctness, the experience of *kumuda* is also possible from the word *pankaja.* It is because of the state of not being correct through *samudāyaśakti,* there arises the understanding on the basis of *lakṣaṇā* of that which grows in the mud.

Reply :

It is not proper to argue that since there is no correctness in the word like *grāmagāma,* there is no *lakṣaṇā,* because with reference to lotus the word *pankaja* is grammatically well-formed.

It is seen that to the usage 'which grows in the mud' correctness means not being produced by illusion. But in the case of *kumuda* it is not a fact. if it is asked we have the following answer. The words like *puṇḍarika* and *navapadma* both express individual understandings.

If somebody asks—that it is the case that we have to accept the knowledge of correctness in each and every sentence which is the cause, it cannot be accepted because, it is impossible to know the state of not being produced by illusion with reference to a new individual sentence and as much there won't be the usage of the word *pācaka* etc. at all.

Objection :

The opponents raise the following doubts—the word *pankaja* is not correct to convey *kumuda* without another *vṛtti* because since there is no *vṛtti* the elderly persons do not use that word to *kumuda*. And whatever word is not used by the elderly persons, those words are not correct without another *vṛtti*. As the word *gangā* is used for bank and *grāmagāma* for 'one who goes to the village', so another *vṛtti* is necessary to convey *kumuda* from the word *pankaja.*

Reply :

It is not tenable, because there is no qualifier worthy to be used since the state of not being used is the pervader. And also because with regard to the sentence having the factors like expectancy etc. and having no correctness, the non-knowledge of the etymological sense in a verbal understanding is proved to be extraneous not approved by the knowledge of grammar and which is the pervader of *sādhya* (probandum). And whatever sentence is grammatically well-formed and possesses expectancy etc. which cause the knowledge of something that sentence is regarded as correct. This statement involves the fault of *satpratipakṣa* and hence the above hypothesis can not be concluded.

And also the knowledge of correctness is not the proper ground because one who knows the etymological sense, even without knowing the earlier usage which is not produced by the illusion etc. uses words in the case of new compositions.

Objection :

How in the case of the word *grāmagāma*, there is no verbal understanding ?

Reply :

Our answer is that it is because of the confirmation of not being correct. And also because in the case of the new literary compositions—there arises no confirmation of the state of not being correct.

Objection :

The opponents put forth another problem that whether there is *śakti* in the suffixes or not ? They argue that whether there is *śakti* in the suffix—*aṇ* which is not followed by the root *gam* or in the suffix *aṇ* other than that which is earlier of the root—*gam* as it is in the form of *kusa-kāśa* being *kuśa* other than that which is earlier of the *kāśa*.

Reply :

It is not possible, because the *śakti* in *aṇ* which is not followed by the root and which is adjacent to a form ending in accusative but not in *aṇ* which is not followed by a root and it is a cumbersome process. And also because when there is no knowledge of specific roots, there does not arise the knowledge of *śakti* and hence there will not arise the usage of such compounds—*kumbhakāra* without knowing the meaning of the *sūtra karmaṇi aṇ* because there is doubt in accepting *śakti.*

The problem arises—whether there is *śakti* to a complex form or not ? The Naiyāyikas say no it is not true, when we listen to a complex word, after listening we remember the individual meanings of the components of that complex form through *śakti.* And in this present context we should not mention the cause and effect relationship by mentioning the individual because in that case there will be multiplicity of cause—and effect relationship. A general rule that—*karmopapadadhātuttarāṇtvena śaktigrahaḥ* will include all cases without any difficulty.

The Naiyāyikas define *asādhutva* as the state of not being correct as per the rules of grammar which is decided by the state of not being acceptable to the elite.

The correctness of a word is *vṛtti* and that is the relation between a word and its meaning and that causes the verbal understanding. The correctness of a sentence means possessing expectany etc. which is expressive of the relation with its word meaning and not being prohibited by the grammatical rules. Hence, even though the word *paṅkaja* is correct, it is not used in the sense of *kumuda* and that is why the *samudāyaśakti* is established.

Objection :

The opponents argue that let the word—*ja* only be treated as having *śakti* but not in the whole word *paṅkaja.* There will be no harm.

Reply :

But the Naiyāyikas answer that it is not proper to argue in the above manner, because there will arise the contingency of the knowledge of lotus in the case of the word like *Manduraja* 'one who is born in a stable', where the word *ja* will have only the expressive power. And if this *śakti* will be accepted in the final member of a word, then in all cases there will be *śakti* in the last letters and hence there won't be any necessity of accepting *samudāyaśakti* at all, which is not true. The Naiyāyikas define *śakti* as that which being known expresses the meaning through some relation.

Gaṅgeśa develops upon his arguments in some cases. He cites the case of the obstruction of the etymological sense. In the case of the word *lambakarṇa*, there should be no obstruction of the etymological sense, because by the inclusion in lotus on the basis of etymology the knowledge of its meaning is possible and hence both the *avayava* and *samudāyaśaktis* are on par.

With regard to the obstruction with the primary relation of the action of bringing—we say that—in the case of the sentence—*paṅkajam ānaya*, the meaning lotus is immediately remembered and is related to the action of bringing, but not to that what grows in the mud, because that is the sentence meaning and hence delayed.

Objection :

If it is said that since there is no contradiction that conventional meaning dominates over the etymological meaning, then ?

Reply :

We say that, it is not justifiable, because it depends on the knowledge of the root and its meaning both by the help of the knowledge of the compatibility etc. and also because the understanding of both the meanings by *yoga* and *rūḍhi.* And hence all the factors after being present immediately appears in the process of verbal understanding. Therefore, the *samudāya-śakti* (*rūḍhi*) is established neither as an obstructor nor the *yoga* is obstructed by it.

Gaṅgesa's Own Arguments

Gaṅgeśa gives his own arguments in favour of *Yogarūḍhi* as a category of words. He puts forth the view that—*rūḍhi* is for the regular remembrance of the meaning lotus and through *rūḍhi* only regularly one uses or experiences the remembered lotus. Through etymology i.e. (*yoga*) *avayavaśakti* 'one experiences that which grows in the mud', because there is a rule that without an obstruction the words expressing the particular individuals stand for the particular meaning which is adjacent to it.

That is why in all cases of the usage of the word *paṅkaja* there arises the experience of lotus through auxiliary factors but the knowledge and the usage do not arise with reference to lily. He emphasizes the arguments of the opponents that—*śakti* is not that which does not cause experience, but *śakti* is that which is known and regularly expresses its meaning.

Both the *avayavaśakti* and the *samudāyaśakti* are the causer of experience, by which the remembrance of meaning is possible. And then *rūḍhi* is also treated as the causer of experience because in the case of the sentence—*paṅkajam ānaya,* both the *avayava* and *samudāyaśakti* are treated as causes.

Hence on the basis of the regular remembrance of the meaning *rūḍhi* is established but not as an obstructor of the primary sense. And if the opponents argue that sometimes the regular remembrance of the meaning is possible through other means, it is surely an instance of *yoga* but not *rūḍhi*. Because with reference to the rule that *yogād-rūḍhirvalīyasī*, with regard to *kumuda* there is no knowledge and usage.

With reference to the opponents view that let the word *go* be treated as *yogarūḍha* category of words. Here, Gaṅgeśa refers to that argument and remarks—that the word *go* stands for cow and the word *ahīna* is used in the sense of a sacrifice conventionally, because it is logically simpler.

One should not argue that from the *uṇādi sūtras gamer doḥ, ahnaḥ khaḥ, kratau dā-bhā-bhyām nuḥ* etc., there is etymology because in ordinary usages the suffixes *ḍa*, *kha* etc. are not used to convey an agent and a particular sacrifice and hence *śakti* is not established here in the suffixes.

But one should postulate the regulating factor in the suffixes nemely—'being subsequent to the root *gam*—and being subsequent to the word—*ahar*. And hence this kind of postulation will certainly lead to cumbersomeness.

To the opponents argument that if the word *go* is not a *yogarūḍha* type of word, let there be *śakti* in the suffix—*nu* in the word *dhenu*, Gaṅgeśa replies—it is not proper because in the word *dhenu*, also, since there is logical inconsistency expresses through *rūḍhi*, that which is an object of milking' and which possesses cowness', because regularly one is reminded of that which possesses *gotva*. So the meaning is not confirmed through etymology also.

So also one cannot postulate *śakti* in the suffix—*nu* in the case of the words like *dānu*, *bhānu* and *kṛsānu* etc. since there is difference in meanings, but by the knowledge of the grammatical rules *gamer ḍoḥ, ahnah khaḥ, kartau dā-bhā-bhyām nuḥ, dheṭa itca* etc., it is necessary to find out the etymological meaning somehow like the word *alavaḍḍa*.

Therefore, the great grammarian Pāṇini has brought those words whose etymology is not possible easily, under the rule *uṇādayo vahulam.* Since the different meanings of such words can not be in one group in comparison to the *samudāyaśakti* enjoined the suffixes which are not enjoined in the *pañcapādıkā* section of the *Aṣṭādhyāyi.* Because there is no *śakti* in *uṇādi* suffixes, where there is *śakti* in the suffix, there he has classed those words to one *sūtra* separately.

Objection :

Here Gaṅgeśa records the views of the *Prābhākaras* (Gurumata that, cowness is not the expressed sense of the word *dhenu,* but merely an *upādhi,* 'an indicatior of the expressed sense'. Where there is cowness, the object of milking and the expressed sense are implied and it is concluded from buffalo etc. and these are brought into one group, since there is unity in indication.

But it is not tenable because one can also say that due to logical simplicity let the cowness be the expressed sense and the object of milking be an *upādhi,* because that cowness which is indicated will lead to the state of over-application and that is logically inconsistent. And also because the remembrance of the object of milking which is qualified by cowness is one and is produced by both a word (cow) and the impression, but not after the remembrance of both. There also arises the verbal understanding of the mutual relationship because there is no *avayavaśakti.*

Reply :

Gaṅgeśa thus replies to the above issue. It is not true in the case of cowness. Because there does not arise the regular remembrance of cowness without *śakti* and also it is proper to say that through the unity of indication, there is unity of indicated. Otherwise, there is no *śakti* in the object of milking excluded from buffalo etc. and both the object of milking and cowness should be the *upādhi* of the *śakti.* And also the understanding arises of the relation of both the object of milking and cowness remembered through impression, the object of milking is also not to be treated as the expressed sense.

If it is said that the consecutive qualifier is the *upādhi* of *śakti* and there is *śakti* with reference to the qualificand and by *upādhi* the meanings could be brought into one group. And hence there will be no contingency of over-application, then there should not be *śakti* with reference to the qualified, in case of the words like *aupādhika—kāraṇa.*

Objection :

Gaṅgeśa again raises the doubt of the opponents that through *avayavaśakti*, there arises the knowledge of 'that which grows in the mud' and through *samudāyaśakti* there will arise the remembrance of lotus from the word *paṅkaja,* but not the experience of lotus which grows in the mud as one which is treated as *yogarūḍha.*

Reply :

It is not true, because the knowledge of lotus which grows in the mud is produced by both *avayava* and *samudāyaśakti* together, as lotus which grows in the mud being remembered by *avayava* anJ *samudāyaśakti.*

And also because the relationship with its meaning is known either by *avayavaśakti* with reference to the lotus which is presented by *samudāyaśakti* or the relationship with its meaning which is experienced through *samudāyaśakti.* With reference to the experience that which grows in the mud which is produced by the *avayavaśakti.* It is because there is a rule that the words having expectancy etc. cause the knowledge of the relationship with their meanings presented by the intention of the speaker.

Gaṅgeśa refers the earlier views of the opponents and refuting that says—it cannot be argued that in other sentences as the knowledge of relationship is not seen, there is no etymology of that type possible. Because in this case on the strength of *samuaāyaśakti* either in the form of a word or a sentence the relationship is known from one expression when presented in both forms. And hence, with reference to both that which grows in the mud and lotus, through *samudāyaśakti* there is sentence unity. But in the sentence—*pankajam kumudam ānaya,* on the basis of *samudāyaśakti* only, 'that which grows in the mud' is not an expressed sense and is indicated by its own meaning which is related to lotus.

Objection :

If it is argued that, since there is correctness in *kumuda,* how there is *lakṣaṇā* in that word ?

Reply :

It is not true, because there will be *asādhutva* with reference to *kumuda.*

Objection :

Here Gaṅgeśa also records the earlier views of the opponents. There was a view that since lotusness is not compatible, it is not related to *kumuda* on the basis of *yoga* i.e. the primary relationship, there arises the knowledge of that which grows in the mud from the word *kumuda.*

Reply :

It is not the case, because the *avayavaśakti* in the word *kumuda* is obstructed by the *samudāyaśakti* which is known and also because that word *kumuda* is known in that manner.

Objection :

The opponents argue that—when by the rule that the word expresses a particular-individual there does not arise the knowledge with reference to *kumuda.* Because, the *avayavaśakti* obstructs it, in such case then the knowledge that arises is that *paṅkajam padmam* from the word *paṅkaja* and since it is not compatible with the sentence meaning by removing *padma* by the sentence unity of a word and sentence. If it is said that, there arises the knowledge of *kumuda* which grows in the mud.

Reply :

Our reply will be in such case we feel there is no need of

taking resort to expectancy of that which grows in the mud which is presented by the relationship with reference to lotus and hence one should accept *lakṣaṇā* for understanding separately for the word *kumuda* as in the case of the word *purodāśakapāla*, the deity is known separately through *lakṣaṇā* only.

Objection :

Again he raises some doubts of the opponents that if it is argued that through the *avayavaśakti*, *kumuda* is compatible with its relationship and having kept aside the remembered meaning lotus, there is the knowledge of its relationship with its own meaning.

Reply :

It is not true, because before the knowledge of the compatibility with its own meaning of the word *kumuda*, since there is earlier knowledge that *paṅkaja* is *padma*, from the word *paṅkaja*, there is no ground of being delayed. And also in the case of the word *sthalapadma* it is treated as of different class, but their is *lakṣaṇā*, while belonging to the same class like *kumuda*.

Objection :

Since there is incompatibility the etymological sense is not known but by compatibility lotusness is conveyed which is presented by *rūḍhi*.

Reply :

It is also not tenable, because lotusness is known by the etymological sense. The secondary relation is necessary in order to have independent remembrance of meaning.

6.0. *ANALYSIS*

It may be observed from whatever is discussed above, that, the terms like *yoga* and *rūḍhi* were used by Pāṇini, Patañjali and Bhartṛhari. Bhartṛhari deals with these terms frequently while discussing the relation between the word and its meaning. He accepts that the meaning lotus is expressed through the conventional relationship from the word *paṅkaja.* Even though he deals with the concepts like *avayava*, *samudāya* and *śakti* but he does not accept *yogarūḍhi* as a separate category of the primary relation over and above *yoga* and *rūḍhi*. Hence the question of accepting *yogarūḍhi* category of words does not arise at all. Among the grammarians the commentator of the *Ma Bhā Pra.* Kaiyaṭa deals with the term directly.

Śavarasvāmīn uses both the terms *yoga* and *rūḍhi* to mean the etymological relation and conventional relation. He also uses the term like *avayavaprasiddhi* and *samudāyaprasiddhi* which are very similar to the Naiyāyikas concept of *avayavaśakti* and *samudāyaśakti.* But he does not use the term *yogarūḍhi* as a separate type of primary relation. The idea of *yogarūḍhi* is very much transparent in the context of the meaning of the term *pratyakṣa* in *Ślokavārttika.*[1] On this, the commentators Sucarita Miśra and Pārthasārathi while discussing the word *śāstra* clearly state that the word *śāstra* is a *yogarūḍha* category of words like the word *paṅkaja* etc. So from their time the word is much used.

But Vāmana and Jayanta Bhaṭṭa quote the opinions of some of the earlier scholars who are in favour of *yogarūḍhi.* But unfortunately, it is not clear whom they are quoting.

For the first time it is Śaśadhara, the pre-Gaṅgeśa author, who presented an analytic essay on *yogarūḍhi* and advanced reasons for its acceptance. The opponents argue that the word *paṅkaja* is expressed in the sense of lotus by the help of *avayavaśakti* and *samudāyaśakti* independently. The earlier is the Grammarian's view and the latter of the Bhāṭṭas.

But Śaśadhara refutes their stands and establishes that it is necessary to accept *yogarūḍhi* over and above *yoga* and *rūḍhi* independently.

Gaṅgeśa deals with all these opponents' views and refutes them. In *Tat. Ci.* we find that those arguments which are given by Śaśadhara have also been taken into consideration. Moreover, Gaṅgeśa develops upon the earlier arguments of Śaśadhara and gives a better reason and clarification in favour of *yogarūḍhi.* At last he has given his own definition and proves that it is a logical necessity to accept a third category of the primary relation called *yogarūḍhi* which will take care of the words like *paṅkaja* etc.

Thus, the entire data tell us the following :

(1) Everybody accepted *yoga* and *rūḍhi.*

(2) Later the concept of *yogarūḍhi* was introduced.

(3) Arguments were presented both in favour of or against the concept of *yogarūḍhi.*

(4) Śaśadhara presented a full picture.

(5) Gaṇgeśa supported Śaśadhara.

(6) Thereafter, almost all schools accepted *yogarūḍhi.*

Notes

1. 1.1.4—130; p. 126.

6.1. *NECESSITY FOR ACCEPTING THE CATEGORY OF YOGARŪḌHI*

It is an observed fact that the words express meanings with the help of different relationships. The relations are either primary or secondary but without that a word does not express anything. We classify words and its relations with reference to its *prayoga*. In other words we observe a particular word being used in a particular sense. How does it happen ? We look at the *prayoga* and start framing rules of their classification. Some words are found used in etymological sense, while others are found in conventional sense. But there are certain words which cannot be classed either in the first group or in the second group. That compels one to accept a third category of words. Such words are—*paṅkaja*, *kṛṣṇasarpa* and *vāsudeva* etc.

If in the case of the word *paṅkaja*, only *yoga* is accepted it will express the meaning of lily, frog and moss etc. i.e. whatever grows in the mud. If only *rūḍhi* is accepted then there will arise the over-application of the term in case of *sthalapadma* the lotus which grows on the ground.

If there is only *rūḍhi* in the case of the word *paṅkaja* then *rūḍhi* will obstruct the application of the etymological relation which has already been accepted with reference to lily.

Hence, neither *yoga* nor *rūḍhi* can express lotus. This is the reason for which the Naiyāyikas accept a third type of primary relation called *yogarūḍhi* which involves both *avayavaśakti* and *samudāyaśakti*. But the *samudāyaśakti* predominates over the *avayavaśakti*. As a result we get a third category of words namely—*yogarūḍha*. *Yogarūḍhi* is, therefore, accepted for excluding some primary meaning and at the same time including some other primary meaning.

6.2. *TYPOLOGY AND CLASSIFICATION OF WORDS IN WESTERN THOUGHT*

Typology :

Typology is a discipline of linguistics that deals with the classification of languages on the basis of the similarity in structures. The approach remains synchronic. Therefore, it can work within a language too. There are four groups of words which come under linguistic typology.[1] They are as follows :

(i) Transparent versus opaque words.

(ii) Generic versus specific words

(iii) Polysemous words

(iv) Homonymous words

Now let us analyse them one by one.

(i) *Transparent versus Opaque words* :

Under typology, the words are generally divided into two major categories namely—transparent and opaque in a particular language. The transparent words are formed by means of a root with prefixes or suffixes. These words are called as motivated words. These words are known immediately from its components. For example—the German word 'Fingerhut' means—'a hat put on a finger.' It is immediately known if one knows the two components. But the opaque words are not easily understandable. In English and French such words are used in a large number. For example—the English word 'thimple' or the French word 'de' are difficult to understand and analyse because they do not contain any clue to their meanings.[2] But it is true that no word is completely transparent or completely opaque.

(ii) *Generic versus Specific Words* :

Some languages are remarkably rich in words with specific meanings, while others prefer to use general terms. French is usually regarded as having generic group of words like 'aller' means 'less in itself', conveys less information and is therefore, more context bound. Whereas German uses mostly specific words like the verbs—gehen, reiten, fahren. In German language, a large scale of prefixes are used in order to specify every aspect of action expressed by the verb, where as in French it is not the case. French will seldom use a derivative, but German have more derivatives.

(iii) *Polysemous Words* :

This is the name given to the use of the same word in two or more distinct meanings. It is a semantic universal inherent in the fundamental structure of language.

(iv) *Homonymous Words* :

In this case one meaning is linked to several names. In old English 'mete' and mētan have converged and become homonymous in Modern English 'meat' and 'to meat' and Latin 'Laudare' and 'locare' have coalesced in the form 'louer' which can mean 'to praise' or 'to hire' or 'to let'. Language rich in short words will obviously have more homonyms than those where longer words are prevalent.

Classification of Words :

Words may be classified in a language on verious parameters —on the basis of their structure, meaning or relation with their meanings. Stephen Ullmann defines meaning as a reciprocal relationship between the name and the sense, which enables one to call up the other.[3] In a language all words are not derivable. They use the term motivation for derivation. And some words which are used in a particular sense come under the class of conventionality. So the vocabulary consist of two major categories namely—(i) conventional and (ii) motivational.

Conventional :

Many of our words are conventional symbols. Their meanings are acquired from early childhood like table etc. All agree that such and such word expresses a particular meaning. There is no derivation or motivation possible in this category of words. This is called conventionality of a word.[4]

Motivational :

This concept refers to the etymological aspect of a word. Etymology was conceived of as the study of the origin of words. This field of semantics deals with the principles of word-structure. Motivation can arise in three cases :—

(i) *Phonetic Motivation*

In this case the former sound is imitated by another sound and so on. For example-cuckoo, splash etc. which are known from their structure itself. These words are also called as onomatopoeia or eco-words.

(ii) *Grammatical or Morphological Motivation*

A word like 'leader' is derived by the English verb to lead and the suffix : er. It is true that the root word and the suffix are themselves conventional, but their combination is motivated. The same also is applied to the compounds 'house-wife', house and wife are both conventional, but housewife is not, the examples like black-bird, ash-tray, motor-way, fellowship are also included in this category.

(iii) *Motivation by Meaning* :

In this case, the figurative usage is taken into consideration. For example, the word bottle-neck is used in the sense of a 'narrow outlet for read traffic'. The word 'bottle' has a meaning and 'neck' has a meaning but when used together means a third thing metaphorically.

Comparison between Indian and Western ways of Classification of words :

What is observed from the above discussion is that: —

(i) To certain extent the Modern Linguistic Classification agrees with the Naiyāyikas classification and to some extent does not.

(ii) The Naiyāyikas classify words in terms of the relationship between a word and its meaning whereas in Western thought they don't classify in terms of relationship.

(iii) The classification on the basis of conventional is comparable to the Naiyāyikas theory of *rūḍha* category of words. The word *go* is conventional and they use the word table which follow the same conventional usage. But the linguistic concept of motivation includes three types out of which the grammatical or morphological theory may be compared to Naiyāyikas *yaugika* class of words like *pācaka* etc.

(iv) The Naiyāyikas accept desire as the primary relationship between a word and its meaning. In Modern Linguistics though motivation ultimately suggests 'desire' it is not treated as a relation in the linguistics tradition.

(v) In Nyāya system the compound forms are expressed with a separate type of relation called *yogarūḍhi* in the case of the words like *paṅkaja* and *kṛṣṇasarpa* etc. But in Modern Linguistics they include it under motivational theory of classification.

(vi) The Naiyāyikas accept four types of primary relation and these relations result into four kinds of words whereas in linguistics they don't have that kind of idea or classification in their semantic analysis.

In western tradition words are classified on different criteria where as in Nyāya tradition the classification is made on logical notion of relation. The former is more concerned with the structure of words, while the latter is more concerned about systematization.

Notes and References

1. See Ullman, Stephen, *Language and Style*, p. 80.
2. I bid. p. 9.
3. *Words and their use*, p. 33
4. *The Principles of Semantics*, p. 83.

7.0. *CONCLUSION*

From whatever we have discussed so far in this present thesis, we can conclude the following :

(1) The Naiyāyikas classify words in terms of the relationship. This relationship is either primary or secondary. And again the primary relation is divided in to four categories namely—(i) *yoga*, (ii) *rūḍhi*, (iii) *yogarūḍhi*, and (iv) *yaugikarūḍhi*. And corresponding to these relations the words are classified in to four, namely—(i) *yaugika*, (ii) *rūḍha*, (iii) *yogarūḍha*, and (iv) *yaugikarūḍha*.

(2) The verbal understanding arises when the factors like *ākāṅkṣā*, *yogyatā*, *sannidhi* and *tātparya* are present. These are not also sufficient factors for the same. Over and above these factors, the relationship has a dominant role to play in the process of verbal understanding. Unless the relationship is known, there won't arise any verbal knowledge.

So it is the logical necessity that one must have the knowledge of relation between a word and its meaning if he wants to invariably remember that meaning from that word.

(3) We classify words and its relations with reference to its *prayoga*. In other words, we observe a particular word being used in a particular sense. If asked how does it happen? Then the answer will be : we look at the *prayoga* and start framing rules of their classification.

(4) If the word *paṅkaja* is treated as a *yaugikaśabda* the etymology of that word will be like this—*paṅkāt jāyate iti*

meaning 'that whatever grows in the mud'. One understands in this stage anything that grows in the mud like lily, frog and moss etc. Here the meaning which grows in the mud includes all things whatever grows in the mud. It has a bigger scope of application.

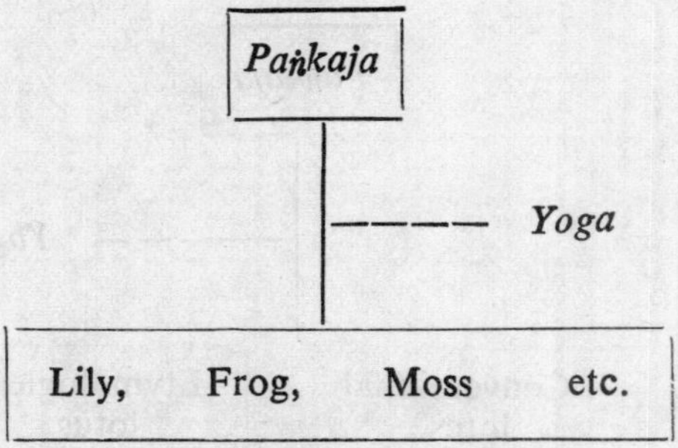

(5) But if the same word *paṅkaja* is accepted through the relation of *rūḍhi* and named as *rūḍha* class of word, then the meaning 'lotus' alone is known through conventional relationship. But the word is also used to mean *sthalapadma*, the 'lotus which grows on the ground'. Thus if *rūḍhi* only is accepted, then it will obstruct the application of the etymological relation which has already been accepted with reference to *sthalapadma*. Thus, it has a limited scope of application.

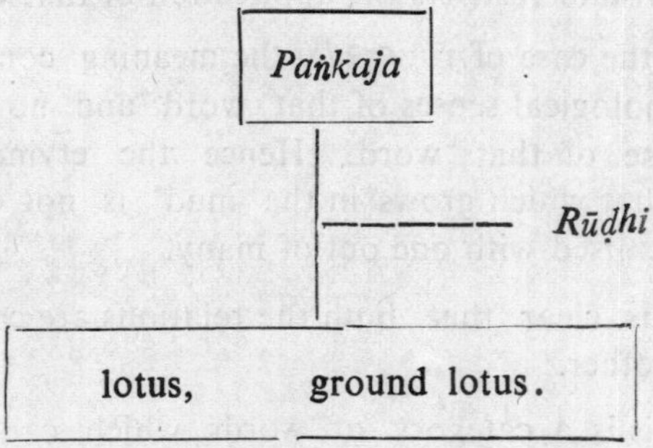

(6) So it is our experience that neither *yoga* nor *rūḍhi* can express lotus from the word *paṅkaja*, for this purpose the Naiyāyikas were left with no other go than to accept a third type of the primary relation called—*yogarūḍhi*. In such a case,

the word *paṅkaja* expresses 'lotus' through *samudāyaśakti* to which *avayavaśakti* is also a helping factor. The conventional relationship is more powerful than the etymological relationship. So the *samudāyaśakti* restricts the application of *avayavaśakti*. There is a wider scope of application of the conventional relationship.

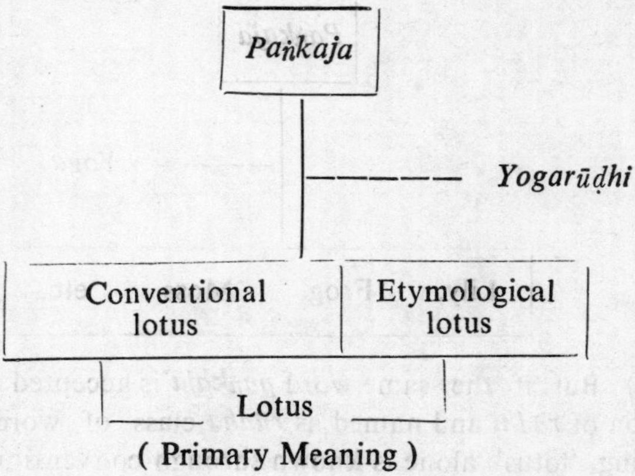

Yogarūḍhi therefore, does the function of both including and excluding both the primary meanings.

(7) The *avayavaśakti* helps the *samudāyaśakti* determine the meaning of the word. The *samudāyaśakti* takes the help of *avayavaśakti* and restricts the application of that word.

(8) In the case of *yogarūḍhi* the meaning conveyed is one of the etymological senses of that word and not any etymological sense of that word. Hence the etymological sense namely—'that which grows in the mud' is not fully ignored but it is localised with one out of many.

(9) It is clear that, both the relations are complimentary to each another.

(10) This is a category of words which can express two meanings but can restrict it to only one.

(11) Neither *yaugika* word nor *rūḍha* word create any ambiguity. It is only *yogarūḍhi* words like *paṅkaja*, *kṛṣṇasarpa* etc. which convey one meaning out of its various possible

etymological meanings. This is the reason that the Naiyāyikas accept a third category of primary relation called *yogarūḍhi*.

(12) In case of the fourth category of relation—*yaugikarūḍhi* both *avayavaśakti* and *samudāyaśakti* are applicable independently. When one is applicable, another is suspended. Both the relations are equally dominant and the meanings are known separately.

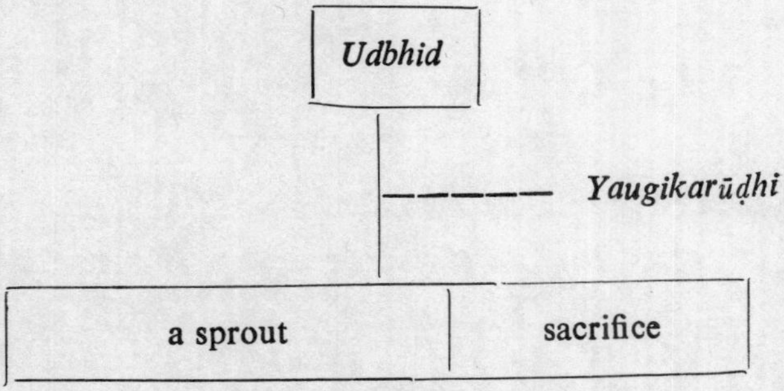

(13) In Indian philosophical analysis, the Mīmāṁsakas, Grammarians, the Naiyāyikas and the Poeticians accept *yoga* and *rūḍhi*.

(14) Later on the concept of *Yogarūḍhi* was introduced before eighth century A.D. The arguments were presented both in favour of or against the concept of *Yogarūḍhi*.

(15) Among the Naiyāyikas, Śaśadhara for the first time critically presented the subject in the form of argumentation. He also for the first time defined the term in Indian Philosophy. Then Gaṅgeśa supported him and improved upon the previous arguments.

(16) After that, we find in all other systems of sentence analysis the concept of *Yogarūḍhi* was accepted as the third type of primary relationship.

This study reveals the parameter on which the classification of words in a language can be based. This has special importance in the context of analysis of verbal epistemology.

Part II

The Yogarūḍhivāda of Gaṅgeśa's Tattvacintāmaṇi

(Text, Translation and Explanatory Notes)

YOGARŪḌHIVĀDAḤ

Original Text, Translation and Explanatory Notes

योगरूढिवादः

TEXT 1

एवं पद्मं पङ्कजपदशक्यं ततो नियमतः पङ्कजनिकर्तृ पद्ममिति प्रतीतेः अवयवानां तत्रासामर्थ्यात् रूढिं विना योगमात्रात् कुमुदे प्रयोगधीप्रसङ्गाच्च।

Translation

Thus, the lotus is the expressed sense of the term *paṅkaja*, because invariably there arises from that term the knowledge such as 'the lotus which grows in the mud'; because the constituents (of the word *paṅkaja*) are not capable to express only on the strength of primary relationship (i.e. *yoga*) that meaning (lotus) without resorting to conventional relationship (i.e. *rūḍhi*). And also because there will arise the contingency of the knowledge of the usage (of the term *paṅkaja*) in the sense of lily (*kumuda*).

TEXT 2

ननु रूढावपि योगात् कुमुदे तौ कुतो न स्यातां रूढ्या-प्रतिबन्धादिति प्राञ्चः।

Translation

Well, even if *rūḍhi* is accepted, why should not there be both the usage and the knowledge, from the primary relationship itself?

(It cannot be) because the conventional relationship obstructs or prevails over the primary relationship, which is the view of the old school.

TEXT 3

वयन्तु नियमतो रूढ्या स्मृतं पद्ममेव व्यक्तिवाचकडप्रत्ययेन पङ्कजनिकर्तृ तयानुभाव्यते बाधकं विना व्यक्तिबचनानां सन्निहितबिशेषपरत्वनियमात् यथाग्नेयीति ढगन्तपदेन प्रकरणादिना सन्निहिता ढगभिहिता ऋग्व्यक्तिर्वोध्यते, एवञ्च सर्व्वत्र पद्मानुभवसामग्र्यैवेति न कुमुदे धीर्न वा तदर्थं प्रयोगः ।

Translation

We, however, hold the view that invariably through convention we remember only lotus from the term *paṅkaja* and through the suffix—*ḍa* which is expressive of individual, we experience it as that which grows in the mud, since it is a rule that the linguistic units expressive of individuals express a particular individual adjacent to it provided there is fact contrary to it.

For example, from the word *Āgneyī* which ends in *ḍhak*-suffix, what is understood is a particular *ṛk* (*mantra*) expressed by the *ḍhak*—and which adjacent to it on the basis of context etc.

Thus, everywhere, there exist the factors which cause the experience of lotus only and hence there is no chance of the knowledge of lily, nor the usage (of the term *paṅkaja*) in that sense.

TEXT 4

नन्वेवं रूढिरेवास्तु तत एवोभयलाभात् किं योगरूढ्या ।

Translation : (Objection)

Well, in that case let there be only conventional relationship because both can be had from that, what is the necessity to accept a third type of relationship called *yogarūḍhi* (i.e. which combines primary and conventional relationship)?

TEXT 5

न अवयवशक्तेः क्लृप्तत्वात् योगिकार्थानुभवाच्च ।

Translation

(Reply) : No. What you say cannot be accepted because the primary relationship is already established (through *avayava-śakti*) and the primary meaning is experienced.

TEXT 6

यदि च रूढ्यर्थं एव यौगिकार्थ एव वानुभूयेत तदा विवादएव न स्यात् अनुभवेनैव तद्विच्छेदात् ।

Translation

If one experiences either conventional sense only or etymological sense only then there won't be any quarrel. Because the difference can be maintained by the knowledge of the experience itself.

TEXT 7

अत्र मीमांसकाः । न तावत् स्मृत्मर्थं शक्तिः पङ्कजपदप्रयोगविषये नियतपद्माधुभवजनितसंस्कारात् स्मृतेरेवोपपत्तेः स्मृतेस्तज्जन्यत्वनियमात् ।

Translation

Here, the Mīmāṁsakas have the following to opine : There is no necessity of positing *Śakti* for the remembrance of the meaning because the remembrance of meaning is possible from the impressions caused by the invariable experience of lotus in the case of the usage of the word *paṅkaja* since a remembrance is invariably caused by an impression.

TEXT 8

नाप्यनुभवार्थं, नियमतः स्मृतं पद्मादाय व्यवितवचनन्यायेनावयवैः पङ्कजनिकर्तृपद्ममित्यनुभवसम्भवात्, स्मृतिश्चरूढ्या अन्यथा वेति न कश्चिदविशेषः ।

Translation

Neither the *Śakti* i.e. the expressive power is required for the experience of that meaning because it is possible to explain the experience of that meaning because it is possible to explain the experience namely 'the lotus that grows in the mud' obtained from the parts (of the word *paṅkaja*) as per the rule that the suffix—*ḍa* which expresses individual. And the remembrance of the meaning can be had either through the conventional relationship or by any other means.

TEXT 9

शक्ति विना नियमतः प्रयोग एव कुत इति चेत् ।

Translation

If it is asked that, without *Śakti* how is the word *paṅkaja* regularly used in the sense of lotus?

TEXT 10

न, पूर्वप्रयोगमपेक्ष्य अवयवानामुक्तन्यायेन पद्मानुभवजनकत्वनियमात् । पूर्वप्रयोगोऽपि तत्पूर्वप्रयोगमपेक्ष्येत्यनादित्व ।

Translation

Our answer is—it is not difficult, because it is invariably seen that the elements of the word *paṅkaja* produce the knowledge of lotus through the suffix—*ḍa* depending upon the earlier usage.

The earlier usage depends upon still earlier usage and hence there will be no end to it.

TEXT 11

अथानियतोद्बोधस्य संस्कारस्य शक्तिं विना नियमोद्बोधे हेत्वभावात् नियता स्मृतिरेव न स्यादितिचेत् ।

Translation

If it is said that since the impression without being regularly stimulated cannot produce regular remembrance and since there is no other regular stimulator other than *Śakti*, there cannot arise regular remembrance.

TEXT 12

य, कदाचिच्छक्तितोऽपि उद्बोधाभावेन शक्यास्मरणात् शक्तिं विनापि नियमतः शक्तिस्मरणाच्च ।

Translation

No, it is not true. Because sometimes it is observed that even though *Śakti* is present the impressions are not stimulated and as a result no remembrance of the meaning takes place and also because even without *Śakti* regularly the remembrance of *Śakti* occurs.

TEXT 13

उद्बोधकञ्च न नियतं सदृशपदशक्तिसम्बन्धिज्ञानानां प्रत्येकं व्यभिचारात्, किन्तु यत्र स्मृतिस्तत्र तत्कालोत्पन्नमनियतमेवोद्बोधकं कल्प्यते फलवलात्, कार्य्योन्नेयधर्म्माणां यथाकार्य्यमुन्नयनात् ।

Translation

Moreover, there is no fixed stimulator possible because it breaks the law of concomitance with the knowledges of similarity, the expressive power of a word and the relatum.

But where there is remembrance a respective stimulator which arises at that time is postulated although that is not any uniform stimulator. This is done on the basis of the effect because the properties which are to be postulated on the basis of an effect are postulated as per each effect.

TEXT 14

न च पद्मत्ववत्तद्व्यापकादेरपि स्मृतिप्रसङ्गः, स्मृतिबलेनोद्बोधकल्पनमिति तत्र स्मृत्यभावेन तदुद्बोधाभावत्, तस्माच्छक्तिं विना शक्तेरिव पद्मत्वस्य नियता स्मृतिः ।

Translation

It is not true to say that there will be contingency of remembrance of the pervader of lotusness (i.e. lily etc.) as of the lotusness. Because a stimulator is postulated on the basis of the remembrance and if there is no remembrance there will be no postulation of any stimulation.

Therefore, without *Śakti* lotusness is regularly remembered as *Śakti* is remembered without *Śakit*.

TEXT 15

न चैवं गवादिपदेऽपि न शक्तिः स्यात् व्यवहारकालीनसंस्कारादेव गवादिस्मृतिसम्भवादिति वाच्यम् ।

Translation

One cannot say that if the argument made above is accepted then, there is no necessity of accepting *Śakti* in the words like *go* 'cow' etc., because on the basis of the impression at the time of usage, the remembrance of the meaning 'cow' etc. is possible.

TEXT 16

न हि तत्र स्मृत्यर्थं शक्तिः, किन्त्वनुभवार्थं पदादन्यतो गवादेरनुभवासम्भवादव्युत्पन्नस्य ततोऽनुभवासम्भवाच्च ।

Translation

(Because) it is not the case that one has accepted *Śakti* for the sake of remembrance (of the meaning 'cow' etc.), that is accepted for causing the experience, because from any source other than the word 'cow' the experience of 'cow' (at that time) is not possible.

And also because the person who does not know the relationship between a word *go* and its meaning 'cow' does not get any verbal knowledge of 'cow'.

TEXT 17

पद्मानुभवश्च योगादेवेति न समुदायो हेतुरन्यथासिद्धत्वात्, अतो नानुभवबलात् समुदाये शक्तिकल्पनम् ।

Translation

And also the knowledge of lotus from the word *paṅkaja* is caused by the help of primary relationship (of the constituent elements of that word) and hence *samudāyaśakti* is not the cause of the knowledge of lotus from the word *paṅkaja* because it can be explained otherwise.

Therefore, it is not true that on the basis of experience one should postulate *samudāyaśakti*.

TEXT 18

नन्वेवं गवादिपदानां प्रमेयत्वे शक्तिरस्तु गवादिस्मृतिः संस्कारादिति चेत् ।

Translation

Well, let the word *go* be expressive of the contentness. The remembrance of 'cow' however, occurs through impression.

TEXT 19

न, गोव्यवहारेण स्वोपपादके गोज्ञाने पदस्य शक्तिकल्पनं न त्वनुपपादके प्रमेयत्वेन गोज्ञाने गोपदात् प्रमेयो गौरित्यननुभवाच्च ।

Translation

It is not proper, because it is necessary to postulate primary relationship with the knowledge of 'cow' which will explain the usage of the word *go*, but not with the knowledge of the content which does not explain such usage. Also, because nobody has any experience of the content of the knowledge from the word *go*.

TEXT 20

अथैवं संस्कारादेव तीरादिस्मृतिसम्भवे गौणलाक्षणिकोच्छेदः, तीराद्यनुभवार्थं हि न तत्कल्पनं तदनुभवस्येतरपदादेव सिद्धेः । तयोरननुभावकत्वात्, तस्मान्नियता स्मृतिः वृतिसाध्येति तयोः कल्पनात् ।

Translation

Well, if it is said that on the basis of impressions alone when the remembrance of 'bank' etc. is possible (in the sentence *gaṅgāyām ghoṣaḥ*) there will arise the contingency not to accept the category of words having secondary relation.

For the experience of the 'bank' one does not postulate that (*lakṣaṇā*), because that experience (of bank) is possible from the other word (in the sentence). Because they both are not capable of generating experience.

Therefore, regularly remembrance is caused by the relationship *vṛtti* (i.e. the relationship between a word and its meaning) and on this basis both the categories are postulated.

TEXT 21

तथाच नियतपद्मस्मृत्यर्थं पङ्कजपदेऽपि वृत्तित्वेन शक्तिकल्पनमावश्यकं लक्षणाद्यभावादिति चेत् ।

Translation

Thus, in order to explain regular remembrance of lotus from the word *paṅkaja* it is necessary to postulate *Śakti* as the primary relationship between a word and its meaning, since there is no *lakṣaṇā* etc.

TEXT 22

न, गङ्गायामित्यादौ वृत्तिं विना तीरादेरपदार्थत्वे विभक्त्यर्थान्वयस्तत्र न स्यात् विभक्तीनां प्रकृत्यर्थगतस्वार्थान्वयबोधकत्वव्युत्पत्तेः । पद्मस्य तु पङ्कजवाक्यप्रतिपाद्यत्वेन पाचकादेरिव विभक्त्यर्थान्वयोपपत्तिः ।

Translation

(Reply): It is not correct, because in the sentence *Gaṅgāyām* (*Ghoṣaḥ*) etc. without a *vṛtti* the meaning 'bank' etc. cannot be treated as word-meaning and as a result the meaning of the case-ending cannot be related to it. Because, there is a rule that the case suffixes cause the understanding of its own meaning connected with the meaning of the word after which they are added. The lotus, however, is conveyed by the sentence (phrase) :*paṅkaja*— it is possible to relate the meaning of the case ending as in the case of *pācaka* 'one who cooks'.

TEXT 23

यतु शब्दोपस्थित एव शाब्दान्वयबोध अन्यथा प्रत्यक्षोपस्थिते कलाये पचतीत्यन्वयबोधः स्यादिति ।

Translation

With regard to the rule that in a verbal understanding the relation of one word-meaning is understood with another word-meaning and if this is not accepted then the meaning of *pacati* will get related to *kalāya* which is perceived by eyes.

TEXT 24

तन्न । पदस्य तत्रतात्पर्याग्रहात् तद्ग्रहे भवत्येव किं पचसीत्युक्ते बधू-पर्दाशतकलायादौ, अन्यथा दैवात् श्रुत-स्मृतकलायपदात् कुतो नान्वयवोधः ।

Translation

But it is not the case, because the speaker does not intend that word in that sense. (And) if he intends, then such relation is indeed possible in the case when someone asks : What are you cooking? and the daughter-in-law shows *kalāya.*

Otherwise, why is such a relation not understood from the word *Kalāya* either heard or remembered by chance ?

TEXT 25

द्वारमित्यादावपि न पिधेहिपदाध्याहारः किन्तु तदर्थस्येवलाघवात् ।

Translation

In the case of the expression *dvāram* (door) also, one does not supply the word *pidhehi* (close), but he supplies only its meaning, since it is logically simpler.

TEXT 26

न च पद्मानयेत्यादौ शाब्दानुभवे पद्मोपस्थापकपदजन्यत्वादन्यत्रापि तथेति वाच्यम् ।

Translation

One need not argue that, since in the understanding arising from the sentence '*padmam ānaya*' the understanding of lotus is caused by the word *padma* and so elsewhere also one should accept the same rule.

TEXT 27

शाब्दपद्‌ानुभवे हि तदन्वयबोधतात्पर्य्यंकपदत्वेन कारणता न तु पद्मो-
पस्थापकपदत्वेनापि गौरवात् ।

Translation

Because for the understanding of the lotus, the word *padma* is the cause as having the intention of the speaker for the understanding of lotus related with bringing but not as a word which presents lotus because it involves cumbersome process.

TEXT 28

अथैवं जनिकाल एवप्रयोगः स्यात् न तदत्ययेऽपि ।

Translation

Well, the word *paṅkaja,* in that case, should be used only when the lotus is being born in mud at a particular moment and cannot be used when that time of growing is over.

TEXT 29

न ह्यसति हि दण्डे दण्डीति व्यपदिश्यत इति चेत् ।

Translation

Because no one uses the word *daṇḍī* 'a man with the staff when there is no *daṇḍa* 'staff present.

TEXT 30

न, पाचकादिपद इव प्रत्ययस्य योग्यताशक्तत्वात् तल्लक्षकत्वाद्वा उपसर्गादौ
तथा निर्णयात्, अन्यथा योगरूढावपि जनिकाल एव प्रयोगः स्यात्, योगत्यागे
केवलरूढिवादे विवादाभावश्च ।

Translation

(Reply) : It is not correct because as in the word *pācaka* cook' in the present case of *paṅkaja* also the suffix is capable of referring to the state of lotus even after the time of the birth of it through primary relationship or through the secondary relationship. This was discussed and we have already taken a decision to that effect while discussing the meaning of *upasargas* earlier.

Otherwise, even in the case of *yogarūḍhi* 'etymologico-conventional sense', one should use the word *paṅkaja* only at the time of its being born. And if one gives up the 'etymological sense' and accepts only 'conventional sense', there is no quarrel with regard to its being only a conventional form.

TEXT 31

तथापि कुमुदे लक्षणा न स्यात् योगार्थस्याबाधादिति चेत् ।

Translation

(If one says that he welcomes it, he cannot say so) because in that case *lakṣaṇā* cannot be applied to obtain the meaning lily from the word *paṅkaja*, because there is no chance of any contradiction with the primary sense.

TEXT 32

न, वक्ष्यते हि तत्र तस्यासाधुत्वम् ।

Translation

(Reply) : This is not proper, we will discuss on this issue afterwards.

TEXT 33

नव्यास्तु नियमतः स्मृतपद्मस्यान्वयानुपपत्त्यनन्तरमेव कुमुदधीरिति न तत्र लक्षणाव्यवहारः ।

Translation

The neo-logicians are of the opinion that regularly when there is incompatibility with the remembered meaning *padma* 'lotus,' there arises, the knowledge of *kumuda* 'lily' and one does not call it *lakṣaṇā*.

TEXT 34

वस्तुतो मुख्यतैव तवापि पद्मत्वस्यायोग्यतया अनन्वये योगादेव कुमुदधीर्न लक्षणयेति ।

Translation

Really speaking it is a case of primary relationship only. Even according to you when *padmatva* has no capacity to relate itself, lily is understood only through primary relation but not through *lakṣaṇā.*

TEXT 35

उच्यते । अस्ति व्युत्पन्नस्य पदज्ञानानन्तरं नियमतोऽन्वयप्रतियोगिस्मृतिरत-स्तद्धेतुसंस्कारोद्बोधकं प्रतिबन्धकं बिना पदज्ञानमेव दृष्टानुविधानत्वादनुगत-त्वाल्लघुत्वाच्च ।

Translation

(Reply): It is the fact that a person who knows the language regularly remembers the meaning which is the counter-relatum of the relation, after he grasps the word and therefore, the knowledge of the word itself, is to be treated as the manifester of the impression if there is no obstacle to do so. Because this is how it is observed in every case and also because it is logically simpler.

TEXT 36

न तु प्रतिपदार्थस्मृतितत्कालोत्पन्नमनन्तमदृष्टचरमनिर्वचनीयं गौरवात् ।

Translation

But not the endless number of unseen inexplicable factors arising at that time, the remembrance of the meaning fro m each word, because it is cumbersome.

TEXT 37

अतः पद्मस्मृतावपि गृहीतसम्बन्धं पङ्कजपदमपि तथेति सम्बन्धत्वेन शक्ति-सिद्धिः ।

Translation

Therefore, with reference to the remembrance of the meaning *padma* 'Lotus' (the knowledge of) the word *paṅkaja* should be taken as the manifester of the impression (leading to the remembrance of the meaning 'lotus'). Therefore, the primary relationship is established as a relation.

TEXT 38

एवञ्च रथकारशब्देऽपि जातिविशेषे रूढिर्न स्यात् संस्कारादेव तदुपस्थित-सम्भवात् तथाच वर्षासु रथकारोऽग्नीनादधीतेत्यत्र रूढयर्थस्य बलवत्त्वेन शीघ्रमुप-स्थितत्वात् जातिविशेषवत एवाधानं विधीयत इति राद्धान्तव्याघातः।

Translation

Thus the word *rathakāra* will not stand for a particular caste conventionally because it is possible to remember that particular caste when the impression will be manifested.

This will lead to the following consequence : In the sentence "in the rainy season the *rathakāra* should perform the *Agnyādhāna* rite, since it is the conventional meaning which is stronger than the etymological meaning (*yogād rūḍhir baliyasī*), the conventional meaning i.e. the particular caste will be presented to the mind (from the word *rathakāra*) quicker, the *ādhāna*—rite is enjoined for the particular caste only. Such a conclusion (of the Mīmāṁsā system) will be contradicted.

TEXT 39

यथाच शाब्दः सन्निधिरन्वयबोधाङ्गं तथोक्तमासतिप्रस्तावे।

Translation

That the proximity of words is the cause of verbal understanding is already discussed while discussing *āsatti.*

TEXT 40

स्यादेतत्, पद्मे नियतप्रयोगरूपसम्बन्धेन पङ्कजपदादेव पद्मस्मृतिरस्तु।

Translation

Perhaps the following is the idea : let one remember lotus from the word *paṅkaja* since there is a relation of the form of regular usage of the word *paṅkaja* to refer to lotus.

TEXT 41

एवञ्च पद्मे विभक्त्यर्थान्वयः शाब्दानुभवप्रवेशश्चोपपद्यते पङ्कजपदप्रति-पाद्यत्वात्।

Translation

And thus the relation of the meaning of the suffix with lotus and its appearance in the verbal understanding become explicable because the understanding is caused by the word *paṅkaja*.

TEXT 42

न च प्रतिपाद्यता वृत्त्यैव तदुपयोगिनी, पाचकमानयेत्यादौ वाक्योपस्थाप्ये तदभावात् ।

Translation

One cannot say that, the relation of the suffix-meaning with lotus and the appearance of the relation in the verbal understanding are helped by the relation between word and meaning because in the sentence *pācakam ānaya* 'bring the cook' there is no *vṛtti* present with reference to that which is presented to our mind by that sentence.

TEXT 43

न च पदाद्वृत्त्यैव स्मृतिः, किन्तु सम्बन्धिज्ञानाद्वृत्तेरपि सम्बन्धत्वे न स्मृत्युपयोगात् अन्यथा पदाच्छक्तेः स्मृतिर्न स्यात्, गवादिपदे त्वेवं स्मृतिसम्भवेऽप्यन्वयानुभवार्थं शक्तिरित्युक्तम् ।

Translation

It is not true that the remembrance (of meaning) is caused by the *padavṛtti* alone but from the knowledge of the relata *vṛtti* helps the remembrance of a meaning as a relation. Otherwise from a word one cannot remember the primary relation.

Although in the word like *go* 'cow' etc. the remembrance is possible, the primary relation (*anubhāvaka śakti*) is accepted for getting the verbal understanding of the relations of word meanings. This is what is stated.

TEXT 44

एतेन पङ्कजपदान्नियमतः पद्मज्ञानं नावृत्तिं विना अतोलक्षणाद्यभावे शक्तिरित्यपास्तम् ।

Translation

Because of such position, the view that since one does not get from the word *paṅkaja* regularly the knowledge ot lotus without *vṛtti* and so there is no need of taking resort to the secondary relation is also refuted.

TEXT 45

ज्ञानं हि स्मृतिरनुभूतिश्च शक्तिं विनाप्युपपन्ना न तां कलपयति अनन्यलभ्यस्यैव शब्दार्थत्वात्, अन्यथा शक्तिं विना पदान्नोपस्थितिरित्यन्वयेऽपि शक्तिर्लक्षणोच्छेदश्च ।

Translation

The knowledge is botn remembrance and experience without *śakti* both are possible and hence they do not cause postulation of *śakti*, because only that can be the word-meaning which is not obtained by any other way than the constituent word of a sentence. Otherwise if this rule is not accepted and if it is held that without *śakti* no remembrance of meaning can take place from any word, then one will have to accept *śakti* in the relation (of word-meanings also which appear in the verbal understanding) and there will arise the contingency of not accepting the secondary relationship at all.

TEXT 46

पङ्कजं पद्ममुच्यत इति प्रसिद्धार्थपदसामानाधिकरण्यात् पद्मस्य ज्ञापकं तत् सिध्यति त तु तच्छक्तम् ।

Translation

Paṅkaja is called *padma*—in this expression since *padma* is coreferential with the word *paṅkaja*, the meaning of which is known, the word *paṅkaja* can be treated as indicator of lotus but not an expressive of *padma*.

TEXT 47

अत एव पङ्कजपदं पद्मशक्तं नियमतस्तत्स्मारकत्वात् पद्मपदवदिति निरस्तम् ।

Translation

This is why, the following inference is turned down : the word *paṅkaja* is expressive of the meaning lotus, because it regularly causes the remembrance of lotus as in the case of the word *padma*.

TEXT 48

शक्तौ व्यभिचारात् अनन्यलभ्यत्वस्य पद्मानुभावकत्वस्य चोपाधित्वाच्चेति ।

Translation

Thus, since there arises the contingency of over application of the primary relationship with reference to *śakti* itself the criteria (1) not being obtained through any other source than the linguistic unit and (2) being the generator of the experience of lotus are extraneous factors.

TEXT 49

उच्यते । नियतपद्मस्मृतेरुक्तसम्बन्धेन पङ्कजपदसाध्यत्वे पद्मवत्तद्व्याप्यव्यापकयोरपि नियमतः स्मृतिप्रसङ्गः ।

Translation

(Reply) : Here is the answer : Since there arises the regular remembrance of *padma* if through the said relation of *vyāpti* one establishes it as being accomplished by the word *paṅkaja*, there will arise the contingency of remembering that which is pervaded by and pervader of *padma*.

TEXT 50

अथ पद्मे प्रयोग एव पद्म एव प्रयोग इति नियतसम्बन्धेन पद्मेतरव्यावृत्तेन पद्मस्यैव पदात् स्मृतिः ।

Translation

Well, since there is only usage in *padma* 'lotus' and usage of *padma* only (of the word *paṅkaja*) by such constant relation, let there be the remembrance of *padma* alone, excluded of things other than *padma* from the word *paṅkaja*.

TEXT 51

न चैवं नियतप्रयोगादेव शक्तिसिद्धिः अनन्यलभ्यस्यैव पदार्थत्वादिति चेत् ।

Translation

It is not proper to say that the primary relation is established by the regular usage, because that alone can be the word-meaning which is not attained by any other means.

TEXT 52

न, तर्हि ज्ञानस्यास्य हेतुत्वे सकलप्रयोगादर्शिनो बहुधा पद्म एव गृहीत-प्रयोगस्य समव्याप्तिज्ञानाभावान्न नियता पद्मस्मृतिः स्यात् स्वरूपसतस्तथात्वे वा अगृहीतपद्मप्रयोगस्यापि ततो नियतपद्मस्मृतिप्रसङ्ग ।

Translation

Well, then the knowledge of the usage will be the probans to establish the probandum. But in that case for one who has not seen each and every case of the usage of the word *paṅkaja* and who has seen the usage a few cases, he will not have the knowledge of the co-extensive invariable concomitance and then he should not have the regular remembrance of *padma*, or even though, it is accepted that (it is not required to be known ane hence) the very usage will cause the inferential cognition, there will arise the contingency that one who has no knowledge of the usage will also have the regular remembrance of lotus.

TEXT 53

अथ यादृशः प्रयोगस्त्वयाशक्तिग्राहकत्वेनाभिमतः स एव पद्मस्मारकोऽस्तु ।

Translation

Well, whatever usage, you have accepted as the generator of the knowledge of *śakti*, let the same be treated as the remembering factor of padma 'lotus'.

TEXT 54

न च पद्मत्वस्येव प्रयोगसमव्याप्तत्वेन गृहीतस्य सौरभादेरुपाधेस्ततः स्मृति-प्रसंङ्गः, तवापि शक्तिग्रहप्रसंङ्गात् ।

Translation

It is not proper to say that, there will arise the contingency remembering the fragrance which is an extraneous factor and which is co-pervasive with the usage like the *padmatva,* because there will arise the contingency of accepting primary relatonship with that.

TEXT 55

तयोस्तुल्यत्वेऽपि शक्तिग्राहकप्रमाणे लाघवादितर्कावतारान्नोपाधौ शक्तिरिति ।

Translation

Although both are at par, since it is logically simpler, with regard to the knowledge which causes the knowledge of primary relationship and since *tarka* can be very well introduced, there will be no *śakti* in *Upādhi.*

TEXT 56

यदि तदा तर्कसहकृत एव शक्तिग्राहकत्वाभिमतः सम्बन्धः पद्मस्मृतिहेतुरस्तु ।

Translation

If it is so, then let the relation which is intended as the cause of the knowledge of *śakti* be the cause of the remembrance of *padma,* assisted by *tarka.*

TEXT 57

तर्काद्यनवतारेऽपि बहुधा गृहीतप्रयोगस्य पद्मस्मृतिदर्शनान्न तथेति चेत्, तर्हि तवापि तर्कं विना शक्तिग्राहकाभावात् कथं पद्मस्मृतिरिति तुल्यम् ।

Translation

But even when there is no *tarka* introduced a person who knows the usage in many places gets the remembrance of *padma* and so that is not so.

In that case for you too without applying *tarka,* there is no factor which can cause the knowledge of *śakti* and then how will there be remembrance of *padma.* Thus both are at par.

TEXT 58

न चैवं तत एव शक्तिग्रहोऽपि स्यात्, अनन्यलभ्यस्यैव शब्दार्थत्वादिति ।

Translation

It cannot be argued that the same will cause the knowledge of *śakti* also, that alone can be the word-meaning which is not obtained by any other way.

TEXT 59

मैवं, एवं गवादिपदेऽपि शक्तिग्राहकत्वाभिमतादेवंविधप्रयोगादेव ज्ञाताद्ग-वादेः स्मृत्यनुभवौ स्यातां किं शक्त्या ।

Translation

It is not so. If that is accepted then even from the word *go* 'cow' etc. there will arise remembrance and verbal experience of cow from the knowledge of the intended usage which causes the knowledge of the *śakti*.

TEXT 60

तस्मात् पदाधीना नियता स्मृतिः शक्तिसाध्या वा नियतसम्बन्धसाध्या वा वृत्तिसाध्या वा, तत्र परिशेषादिह शक्तिसाध्यैव ।

Translation

Therefore, the question is whether one should establish regular remembrance of a meaning from a particular word on the basis of primary relation or on the basis of regular relation or on the basis of *vṛtti* ?

From these alternatives the remembrance is possible on the basis of *śakti* only through the method of exclusion.

TEXT 61

न च शक्तिस्मृतौ व्यभिचारः, शक्तिस्मारकत्वाभिमताद्धिपदात् पदार्थ-स्यैवाहत्य स्मरणं न शक्तेर्हेत्वभावात् कल्पनागौरवाच्च सम्बन्धिनं विना सम्बन्ध-स्यास्मरणेन प्रथमं पदार्थस्मरणस्यावश्यकत्वाच्च ।

Translation

There is no violation of this rule with reference to the

remembering of *śakti* because from the word which is intended to be the rememberer of *śakti* the word-meaning alone is remembered, and not the *śakti* because there is no ground for that and also because it will involve cumbersome postulation and also because without the remembrance of the relata the remembrance of relation is not possible, therefore, it is necessary to remember the meaning first.

TEXT 62

पदार्थस्मृतेश्च शक्तिविषयत्वे मानाभावात् उद्बुद्धसंस्कारविषयत्वाद् यदि शक्तिरपि तद्विषयः, तथापि पदार्थशक्तत्वेनैव ज्ञातस्य पदस्य शक्तिस्मारकता न तु शक्तिसम्बन्धित्वेन अन्यथासिद्धत्वात् ।

Translation

There is no ground to hold that the relation also forms part of the content of the remembrance of the meaning.

If *śakti* is to be accepted as the content of that because of the manifestation of the impression, still the word which is known as being capable of reminding its meaning has the capacity to remind but not as merely being associated with *śakti*, since that is established otherwise.

TEXT 63

यद्वा पदान्नियमतः स्मृतिर्न्नियतसम्बन्धसाध्या शक्त्यापि समं पदस्य शक्त्याश्रयत्वमेव नियतः सम्बन्धः ।

Translation

Or, another argument may be as follows : regular remembrance from a particular word is caused by the knowledge of a regular relation and even with *śakti* the word is regularly related as being the locus of that *śakti.*

TEXT 64

अपिच कुमुदेऽवयवशक्तिप्रतिबन्धार्थं रूढ़िः ।

Translation

And there is *rūḍhi* 'conventional sense' (i.e. *samudāyaśakti*) in the whole word *paṅkaja* for obstructing the *śakti* in its components for remembering lily.

TEXT 65

न च नियतपद्मस्मृतिरेव प्रतिबन्धिका, रूढ़िं बिना नियतस्मृतेरभावात् ।

Translation

One cannot argue that the regular remembrance of lotus only is the obstructing factor because without the conventional sense, there is the absence of regular remembrance.

TEXT 66

अत एव न व्यक्तिवचनन्यायोऽपि ।

Translation

This is the reason that the rule of the reference to individual is also not accepted.

TEXT 67

नचैकं पदमेकदैकेनैव रूपेण प्रवर्त्तते अतो न पद्मत्वपङ्कजत्वयोर्धीरिति वाच्यम् ।

Translation

It is also not proper to argue that since a particular word is used once in one sense only and so there will not arise the knowledge of *padmatva* and *paṅkajatva* simultaneously.

TEXT 68

अवयवसमुदाययोर्भेदात् लम्बकर्णादिपदे व्यभिचाराच्च ।

Translation

Because of the difference maintained in both *avayavaśakti* 'relation with constituent and *samudāyaśakti*' 'relation with whole word' and also because in the word like *lambakarṇa* 'one who has a long ear', there will not take place the knowledge of conventional sense.

TEXT 69

तर्हि तद्वदेव रूढ्यानावयवशक्तिप्रतिबन्ध इति चेत् ।

Translation

In that case like that word *lambakarṇa* the *rūḍhi* cannot set aside the *avayavaśakti.*

TEXT 70

न, तत्रावयवार्थक्रियान्वयेनाप्रतिबन्धान्नानार्थे च नानार्थानुभवात् नैक-शक्त्यान्यशक्तिप्रतिबन्धः ।

Translation

It is not true because there (in the word *lambakarṇa*) there is no obstruction but with the action of bringing conveyed through primary relation, there is no obstruction and in the case of polysemus word, many meanings are experienced and so one should accept that one *śakti* is not obstructed by the other.

TEXT 71

यत्तु अवयवशक्तिस्मृतिकाले समुदायशक्तिस्मृतिनियमे हेत्वभावान्न तया प्रतिबन्ध इति ।

Translation

The argument that at the time of remembrance of the *avayavaśakti*, there is no ground that invariably there will be remembrance of *samudāyaśakti* and hence that remembrance will obstruct the remembrance through the *avayavaśakti.*

TEXT 72

तन्न । समुदायस्य तावदवयवरूपत्वेन सर्वावयवादेवोभयशक्तिस्मृतिसम्भवात् मण्डपपदे तथा दर्शनात् ।

Translation

It is not tenable. Because whole is identical with parts and so from the whole the remembrance of both the relations is possible as it is observed in the word *maṇḍapa* (i) one who drinks gruel and (ii) a pandel.

TFXT 73

अथपङ्कोत्तरजपदं प्रतिबन्धकं गोबलीवर्दवत् पङ्कजनिपदप्रयोगे डप्रत्ययस्य

कर्तृविशेषपद्मपरत्वं वा जनेः पद्मजनिविशेषपरत्वं वा स्वभावादेव कुमुदबोधा-जनकत्वं वा चक्षुष इव रसे कुमुदेऽवयवशक्तिकुण्टनं वा कल्प्यतां तेन कुमुदे न धीरिति चेत्, तर्ह्यज्ञातपद्मप्रयोगस्य कुमुदसाधारणबोधो न स्यात् ।

Translation

Well, the constituent word—*ja*—is the obstructor which follows the word *paṅka* as it is in the case of the compound word *go-valīvarda* where the second member obstructs the knowledge of the first one. In the usage of the word *paṅkajani* the *ḍa* (a) suffix refers to a particular agent namely, *padma* 'lotus' or the constituent word *jani*—means a particular growing of lotus or by its nature *kumuda* 'lily' is not conveyed from the word *paṅkaja* or one should postulate the restriction of *avayavaśakti* in the word *paṅkaja* in order to convey *kumuda* as it is observed that through the eyes one does not get the knowledge of taste, and this is how one will not have the remembrance of *kumuda* 'lily' from the usage of the word *paṅkaja.*

TEXT 74

न भवत्येवेति चेत्, किमवयवव्युत्पन्नस्य ततोऽर्थप्रत्यय एव न भवति ।

Translation

Indeed there does not arise the common experience of *kumuda* etc. from the word *paṅkaja.* In that case, two questions arise in one's mind : (1) Is it that a person who knows the etymological sense does not get knowledge from that word ?

TEXT 75

यद्वापङ्कजत्वेन पद्ममेवानुभूयते, आद्ये मन्दुरजादिपदादिव सामग्रीसत्वे कथं नानुभवः ।

Translation

Or (2) Is it that lotus is experienced as that which grows in the mud ?

As regards the first question, how is it that from the word *paṅkaja* an experience does not arise when all factors as in the case of the word *manduraja,* 'one who is born in a stable' ?

TEXT 76

द्वितीये कुमुदमप्यनुभूयेताविशेषात् ।

Translation

In the second case *kumuda* also should be remembered because there is no difference.

TEXT 77

न चैवं पंकजशब्दस्य सामान्यशब्दत्वात् तात्पर्यवशेन विशेषतः पद्मकुमुद-धीसम्भवात् न रूढिर्न वा लक्षणा स्यादिति वाच्यम् ।

Translation

One can not argue that, because the word *paṅkaja* is a common term, and on the basis of the particular intention of the speaker the knowledges of lotus and lily are possible from that word and hence there is no need of conventional or secondary relation.

TEXT 78

न हि प्रयोजनक्षतिभयेन सामग्री नानुभावयति ।

Translation

It is not the case that, because of loss of purpose the factors do not cause the experience.

TEXT 79

यदि च पद्मकुमुदयोस्तुल्यता तदा अगृहीतपद्मप्रमोगस्य पद्मान्वयानुपपत्ति-पुरःसरेव कुमुदधीर्न स्यात् ।

Translation

If it is accepted that both *padma* and *kumuda* are on par, then one who has not seen the usage of *paṅkaja* for 'lily' then on account of impossibility of relation with *padma* there will not arise the knowledge of *kumuda*.

TEXT 80

स्याच्च कदाचिद्वैपरीत्यम् अतः पद्मे रूढिरेव, कुमुदे यथा लक्षणा तथा वक्षामः ।

Translation

And sometimes the reverse may also happen. That is why there is *rūḍhi* in *padma*.

That there is *lakṣaṇā* in *kumuda* we shall discuss later.

TEXT 81

कुण्टनञ्च शक्तिवृत्तिधर्मान्तरं वा शक्तेरनुद्भवो वा अभिभवो वा तत्र कारणान्तरं वा अदृष्टचरं कल्प्यम् ।

Translation

What is restriction may be another property in the *śakti* or non-manifestation of *śakti* or over-powering of *śakti* or some other reason or one might postulate an unseen cause.

TEXT 82

रूढेः प्रयोगप्रतिबन्धकत्वं मण्डपादौ दृष्टमेव ।

Translation

We have already observed how *rūḍhi* obstructs the usage while discussing the word *maṇḍapa*.

TEXT 83

अतएव पंकाद्यवयवैः पद्ममेवानुभाव्यत इति, अवयवनियमस्य कल्पनान्न कुमुदे धीप्रयोगौ ।

Translation

Therefore, from the components *paṅka*, etc., one experiences lotus only and since we have postulated the restriction in the *avayavaśakti*, there does not arise the usage and the knowledge of *kumuda*.

TEXT 84

अन्यथा रूढावपि योगान्न कुतस्तौ कुमुदे, यथा उद्भित्पदस्यऽयोगात् खनित्रे रूढ्या कर्मविशेषे प्रयोग इति निरस्तम् । अगृहीतनियतपद्मप्रयोगस्य कुमुदसाधारणबोधदर्शनात् ।

Translation

Otherwise, in *rūḍhi* also, because of the etymology why

there is no usage and the knowledge of *kumuda* as it is in the word *udbhid*, on the basis of etymology, it is used in the sense of a spade and on the basis of *rūḍhi* one uses it in the sense of a particular rite. Thus it is ruled out.

Because one who does not know regular usage of the word *paṅkaja* to lotus gets the common experience of *kumuda.*

TEXT 85

रूढिवादे तु सैव प्रतिबन्धिका मण्डपपदवत् ।

Translation

But in the rule that *yogād rūḍhirvalīyasī*, that *rūḍhi* itself is the obstructor as in the case of the word *maṇḍapa* 'one who drinks gruel'.

TEXT 86

ज्ञातस्य चावयवनियमस्य प्रयोजकत्वे पद्मे शक्तिरेव पद्मज्ञानजनकत्व-ज्ञानस्य शक्तिनिर्वाह्यत्वात् ।

Translation

And if one accepts the restriction of the primary relation of the components and if that is treated as the causing factor, then let us accept *śakti* (in the word *paṅkaja*) to refer *padma* because the knowledge that generates the knowledge of the *padma* is regulated by *śakti.*

TEXT 87

उद्भित्पदे त्ववयवार्थः कर्मण्ययोग्यत्वादेव नान्वीयते न तु रूढ्या प्रति-बन्धात् ।

Translation

As in the case of the word *udbhid*, however the meaning of the component is not fit to be related to a particular rite and it is not true that the etymological sense is obstructed by the conventional sense.

TEXT 88

अवयवान्वययोग्ये खनित्रेऽपि न प्रतिबन्धः योगेन खनित्रेऽपि प्रयोगात् ।

Translation

Similarly, when the etymological sense is related to a spade, there is no obstruction because on the basis of primary relation the word *udbhid* is used in the sense of a spade.

TEXT 89

एवञ्च रूढियोगाभ्यामुद्भि त्पदस्य नानार्थतुल्यतैव उभाभ्यामेकार्थानवगमात् ।

Translation

And thus both from the conventional and etymological sense, the word *udbhid* will be treated as similar to a polysemous word because both do not convey a single meaning.

TEXT 90

ननु गृहीतपद्मप्रयोगस्यावयवैः सह प्रयोगे पद्ममेवानुभाव्यत इति स्वभावकल्पनमस्तु ।

Translation

Well, one who knows the relationship of the usage of the word *paṅkaja* to lotus, it is observed that the usage causes the knowledge of lotus only and so let us postulate the nature of the word *paṅkaja* to convey lotus.

TEXT 91

नचैवं व्युपत्त्यन्तरं, स्वरूपसत एव प्रयोगग्रहस्य शक्तिग्रहस्येवोपसन्धानत्वात् ।

Translation

This does not involve another etymology because by the very nature itself the knowledge of the usage like the knowledge of the relationship is possible to be the auxiliary factor.

TEXT 92

उपसर्गस्येव धातोः प्रकर्षादिबोधकत्वे, उपसन्धानं विना कुमुदबोधो भवत्येव ।

Translation

As the root-meaning is changed with the nearness of the use of the prefixes to convey the knowledge of excelling etc. are possible and since without the auxiliary factor the understanding of *kumuda* does take place.

TEXT 93

यत्तु पदानां स्वार्थान्वयबोधसामर्थ्यं उपजीव्य कुमुदाबोधार्थं नान्विताभिधानेऽवयवनियमः कल्प्यते, उपजीव्यविरोधात्, किन्तु समुदायस्य कुमुदे स्वार्थत्वाभाव एवेति ।

Translation

The following view is also not tenable. Because the words are capable of expressing their meanings related with other meanings and on the basis of that, for the non-knowledge of *kumuda*, one should not postulate the restriction of the rule in *anvītābhidhānavāda* because of the contradiction of the causal factor, but from *samudāyaśakti* i.e. *rūḍhi* the absence of being its meaning with reference to *kumuda.*

TEXT 94

तन्न । एवं स्वार्थत्वाभावेन समुदायात् कुमुदधीर्न स्यात् अवयवेभ्यस्तु स्यादेवेति ।

Translation

(It is not tenable), because of its not being the primary meaning from *samudāya*, there will not arise the knowledge of *kumuda*, but from components the understanding will definitely take place.

TEXT 95

मैवं । न हि पदानां स्वभावाधीनं बोधकत्वं किन्तु शक्तिज्ञानाधीनमज्ञातशक्तेरबोधकत्वाच्छक्तिभ्रमेण बोधकत्वाच्च ।

Translation

(*Reply*) : It is not acceptable. Because it is not the case that the understanding of meaning depends upon the nature of words but it depends upon the knowledge of the relationship because when the relationship is not known no one understands from a word and also because one understands because of illusory relationship.

TEET 96

तथाच बोधकशक्त्यभावादेवाबोधकत्वं कार्याभावे हेत्वभावस्यैव तन्त्रत्वात् ।

Translation

Thus, because there is expressive relation there is no understanding as per the rule that when there is no effect implies that there is no cause.

TEET 97

धातोश्चोपसर्गोपसन्धानात् प्रकर्षादौ शक्तिरेव ।

Translation

The roots with the auxiliary nearness of the prefixes express excellence through primary relationship.

TEXT 98

स्यादेतत् । यथा सर्वनामत्वमहम्पदेषु बुद्धिस्थत्वसम्बोध्यत्वोच्चारयितृत्वानि प्रयोगोपाधयस्तेन बुद्धिस्थादिकमेव तद्बोधयति ।

Translation

It may be the following: as in the pronoun *aham* 'I' etc. the state of being in the mind, being the object of address and being the speaker are the prompting factors of usage and therefore, that word *aham* refers to that person who is in the mind.

TEXT 99

तत्रैव प्रयुज्यते च न तु बुद्धिस्थत्वादिकं शक्यं तेन रूपेण ज्ञानाभावात् तथा पद्मत्वमपि प्रयोगोपाधिरिति चेत् ।

Translation

And the word *aham* is used to that person only but that being in the mind etc. is not the expressed sense of the pronoun *aham*.

Because from the word *aham* the knowledge of those factors does not arise. Likewise, let lotusness be treated as a prompting factor.

TEXT 100

न, तेन हि नावयवशक्तिर्विच्छिद्यते पद्मे तत्सत्त्वात् ।

Translation

(Reply). It is not tenable, because by that the *avayavaśakti* is not restricted as the word *paṅkaja* refers to lotus through the etymological sense also.

TEXT 101

नापि कुमुदे तात्पर्यमपोद्यते, बाधकं विना तस्यौत्सर्गिकत्वात् ।

Translation

The intention to lily is also not ruled out, because without the obstructor the understanding in general will occur.

TEXT 102

नाप्यवयवाधीनज्ञानं प्रतिबध्यते शक्त्याकांक्षादितात्पर्याणां सत्वे अन्वयज्ञानस्यावश्यकत्वात् उपाधेरन्वयबोधप्रतिबन्धाहेतुत्वात् ।

Translation

The knowledge based on the *avayavaśakti* is not contradicted, because if there are factors like *śakti*, expectancy and the intention of the speaker etc., the verbal understanding necessarily takes place and an extraneous fact is not the cause of the obstructing factor of the verbal understanding.

TEXT 103

नापि प्रयोगो वार्यते, इष्टकुमुदधीहेतुतया इष्टसाधनताज्ञनस्य तल्लिङ्गक कार्यताज्ञानस्य वा प्रयोगहेतोः सत्त्वे अप्रयोगस्याहेतुत्वात् ।

The usage also is not obstructed, because when there is the ground of usage namely the knowledge of *iṣṭasādhanatā* 'being the instrument to obtain the desired object' aiming at knowing the desired lily, or the knowledge of being the volition inferred on that ground the non-usage cannot be the ground.

TEXT 104

अहमादिपदे त्वात्ममात्रशक्तेः शक्तिग्रहसहकारितया स्वरूपसदेव उच्चारयितृत्वादिकं धीनियामकं स्वभावान्नियमतस्तस्यैव बोधनादिति स्वरूपसत एवोपाधित्वम् । पद्मत्वन्तु न तथा, कुमुदसाधारणबोधदर्शनात् ।

Translation

In the words like *aham* 'I' the self only is the expressed meaning and taking the knowledge of the relationship as the auxiliary cause, by its nature only the state of being an utterer regulates the verbal understanding and also because of the very nature itself regularly that pronoun causes the knowledge and hence by itself (nature), *uccārayitṛtva* is *upādhi*.

But it is not the case with lotus-ness, because the common experience of *kumuda* and lotus is an observed fact.

TEXT 105

ननु कुमुदे पूर्वेषामप्रयोगादाधुनिकनामप्रयोगः ।

Translation

Well, if it is argued that, since *paṅkaja* is not used earlier in the sense of *kumuda*, so there is no later usage in that sense.

TEXT 106

न च प्रयोगमात्रे कोहेतुरिति वाच्यम् ।

Translation

It is not proper, because one need not ask : for an usage in general what is the real ground ?

TEXT 107

प्रयोगाणां हि न मेलनकार्यता किन्तु प्रत्येकं, तत्रोत्तरस्य पूर्वहेतुः यथा पूर्वगौरुत्तरस्य अन्यथा गोमात्रे कोहेतुरित्यत्र किमुत्तरं तवेति चेत् ।

Translation

For usage is not caused by an assemblage (of usage) but it occurs individually. To the later usage, the earlier usage is the ground like the earlier usage of the word *go* 'cow' for the later usage. Otherwise, to the usage 'cow' what is the ground if asked by someone in such case, what would be your reply ?

TEXT 108

न, प्रयोगहेतोः सत्त्वात् पूर्वप्रयोगस्य चाहेतुत्वात् पूर्वप्रयोगमज्ञात्वाप्यवयव-

व्युत्पन्नेन पाचकादिपदानां नवकाव्यानां गौणलाक्षणिकदेवदत्तादिपदानां च प्रयोगात् ।

Translation

It is not so, because there is ground for usage and the earlier usage is not the ground because without the knowledge of the earlier usage also the person who knows the *avayavaśakti* (component parts) in the words like *pācaka* etc. new literary compositions, and in the words like *gauṇa*, *lākṣaṇika* and Devadatta etc., there arises the perfect usage.

TEXT 109

स्यादेतत्, ग्रामगामादिपदेऽन्वयबोधाभावात् साधुत्वज्ञानमपि हेतुः ।

Translation

It may be the following : but in the word *grāmagāma*, 'one who goes to a village' since there is no understanding, the knowledge of the correctness also should be the ground.

TEXT 110

न चैवं तदेव हेतुरस्तु किं शक्त्या गौणलाक्षणिकविवेकश्च सोपाधित्वानुपाधित्वाभ्यामेवास्तु इति वाच्यम् ।

Translation

One cannot argue that let that knowledge of correctness be the ground for understanding, what is the necessity of accepting *śakti* and let the knowledge of distinction between *gauṇa* and *lākṣaṇika* be maintained on the basis of being an *upādhi* and not being an *upādhi*.

TEXT 111

प्रथमं व्यवहारेण शब्दस्य ज्ञानकारणतावगमात् तत्रैव शक्तिकल्पनं ततो ग्रामगामादौ व्यभिचारादाकांक्षादेरिव साधुत्वज्ञानस्य हेतुत्वकल्पनात् ।

Translation

Because, by the first usage, the knowledge of the word becomes the cause, and therefore in that word one postulates *śakti* and since in the word *grāmagāma* etc. there is logical inconsistency and like the expectancy etc., one postulates the knowledge of correctness as the cause.

TEXT 112

साधुत्वंच न पूर्वप्रयोगप्रवाहाविच्छेदः नवकाव्यादौ तदभावात्, किन्तु भ्रमादिजन्यत्वाभावः। कुमुदे च ततप्रयोगोबोधकत्वभ्रमात्।

Translation

The correctness is not the continuity of the earlier usage, because it is absent in the new compositions etc., but correctness means absence of being produced by illusion (of relationship) also.

In *kumuda* however, because of the illusion of the relationship, that usage (of the word *paṅkaja*) is found.

TEXT 113

न चैवं भ्रमजन्यत्वादबोधकत्वमबोधकत्वे च भ्रमजन्यत्वमित्यन्योन्याश्रयः।

Translation

It cannot be argued that since there is the state of being produced by illusion, there is the state of not causing understanding and since there is the state of not causing the understanding there is the state of being produced by illusion, which leads to the fault of mutual dependency.

TEXT 114

पूर्वभ्रमजन्यत्वेनोत्तरं प्रति बोधकत्वभ्रमात् उत्तरस्य प्रयोगोभ्रमजन्यः, एवं पूर्वस्यापीति तत्र भ्रमपरम्परैव मूलमेवं ग्रामगामादेरपि।

Translation

Then because of the state of being produced by earlier illusion becomes the cause of the later illusion and hence the later usage is an illusion.

Similarly, the earlier illusion also and thus there starts the chain of illusions which is the main source and like that it is the case with the usage of the word *grāmagāma* etc.

TEXT 115

कथमिदं ज्ञातव्यमिति चेत्।

Translation

How that is known if asked by someone.

TEXT 116

ग्रामगमनकर्त्तरि ग्रामगामपदस्यैव प्रामाणिकानां कुमुदे तस्य निरुपाधि-प्रयोगाभावात् ।

Translation

The answer is that as one understands 'one who is going to the village' from the word *grāmagāma*, a authoritative person do not use the word *paṅkaja* with reference to *kumuda* without any extraneous factor.

TEXT 117

अतएव साधुत्वभ्रमात् कुमुदसाधारणोबोधोऽपि ।

Translation

This is the reason that, because of the illusion of the correctness (factor), the common experience of *kumuda* is also possible from the word *paṅkaja*.

TFXT 118

कुमुदे ह्यसाधुत्वात् समुदायेन तत्र पंकजन्मकर्त्तृत्वं लक्षते ।

Translation

Because of the state of being not correct through *samudāya-śakti*, there arises the understanding through *lakṣaṇā* of that which grows in the mud.

TEXT 119

न चासाधुत्वे ग्रामगामपदवत् लक्षणापि न स्यात्, पद्मे तस्य साधुत्वात् ।

Translation

One cannot argue that, since there is no correctness in the word like *grāmagāma*, there will not be *lakṣaṇā*, because with reference to lotus the word *paṅkaja* is grammatically well formed.

TEXT 120

उच्यते । पंकजन्मकर्त्तरि तत्प्रयोगस्य भ्रमाद्यजन्यत्वेन साधुत्वम् । कुमुदे न तथेति चेत् ।

Translation

Thus it can be answered in the following manner :

To that usage, 'that what is grown in the mud, correctness means not being produced by illusion. But in *kumuda*, that is not the case, if asked by someone.

TEXT 121

न पुण्डरीकवन्नवपद्मवच्च तस्य व्यक्तिस्थानीयत्वात् ।

Translation

Then the answer is, it is not so because like the word *puṇḍarīka* and *nava-padma* as both express individuality.

TEXT 122

प्रतिवाक्यार्थञ्च साधुत्वज्ञानस्य हेतुत्वे अभिनवव्यक्तौ भ्रमाद्यजन्यत्वस्यग्रहीतुमशक्यतया पाचकादिपदप्रयोगो न स्यात्, पाककर्तृजातीये भ्रमाद्यजन्यत्वस्य सुग्रहत्ववत् पंकजन्मकर्तृजातीयेऽपि सुग्रहत्वात् येन रूपेणान्वयबोधस्तस्य कुमुदवृत्तित्वात् ।

Translation

If to each individual sentence meaning the knowledge of correctness is required as cause since it is impossible to know the state of not being produced by illusion with reference to a new individual, there will not be the usage of the word *pācaka* etc. Because, as in the class of one who cooks, it is possible to know the state of not being produced and similarly, it is possible to know the same with reference to 'that which grows in the mud' and the form in which verbal understanding arises that is present in *kumuda*.

TEXT 123

अथ पंकजपदं कुमुदे वृत्त्यन्तरं विना न साधुवृत्त्यन्तरं विना वृद्धैस्तत्राप्रयुज्यमानत्वात्, यः शब्दो यत्र वृत्त्यन्तरं विना वृद्धैर्न प्रयुज्यते स तत्र वृत्त्यन्तरं

विना न साधुः यथा गङ्गापदं तीरे, यथा वा ग्रामगामपदं ग्रामगमनकर्त्तरि, न प्रयुज्यते च वृत्त्यन्तरं विना पंकजपदं कुमुदे तस्माद्वृत्त्यन्तरं विना न तत्र साध्विति चेत्।

Translation

Well, the word *paṅkaja* is not correct to convey *kumuda* without another *vṛtti*, because without another *vṛtti*, there is no usage by the elderly person (of that word) to *kumuda*; whatever word is not used by the elderly person without another *vṛtti*, that word is not correct without another *vṛtti* with reference to that meaning as the word *gaṅgā* stands for the bank (through *lakṣaṇā*) and as the word *grāmagāma* is used in the sense of that one who goes to a village, And without another *vṛtti* the word *paṅkaja* is not used for *kumuda*.

Therefore, without another *vṛtti*, it is not correct (to convey *kumuda*).

TEXT 124

न, व्यर्थविशेषणत्वात् तत्राप्रयुज्यमानत्वस्यैव व्याप्यत्वात् आकांक्षादिमद्वाक्यासाधुत्वे अवयवार्थान्वयाबोधकत्वस्य व्याकरणस्मृत्यनुपगृहीतत्वस्य पक्षधर्मावच्छिन्नसाध्यव्यापकस्योपाधित्वाच्च।

Translation

(Reply) : It is not the case, because the qualification is futile since the state of not being used is the pervaded (probans). And also because, with regard to the sentences, having expectancy etc. and having no correctness, the non-knowledge of the etymological sense in a verbal understanding is proved to be extraneous, not approved by the knowledge of grammar and which is the pervader of *sādhya* (probandum).

TEXT 125

पक्षे उभयाभावेन साधनाव्यापकत्वात्। पंकजशब्दः कुमुदे साधुः साधुत्वे सति कुमुदबोधप्रयोजकाकांक्षादिमद्वाक्यत्वात्, साधुत्वे सति यद्वाक्यं यद्बोधप्रयोजकाकांक्षादिमद्भवति तत्तत्र साधु यथा तरूप्रसूनशब्दः कुसुमे, यथा वा पाचकशब्दः पाककर्त्तरि, तथा पंकजपदं कुमुदे तस्मातथेति सत्प्रतिपक्षत्वाच्च।

Translation

Since there is *ubhayābhāva* in *pakṣa* it is not the pervader of the *hetu.* (As against this) The word *paṅkaja* is correctly used in the sense of *kumuda*, because it is grammatically well formed and it is a sentence which has expectancy etc. which cause the knowledge of *kumuda*.

And whatever sentence is grammatically well-formed and possesses expectancy etc. which cause the knowledge of something that sentence is regarded to be correct with reference to that thing like the word *tarūprasūna* is used in the sense of a flower, or as the word *pācaka* is used in the sense of that 'one cooks' like that the word *paṅkaja* is used in the sense of *kumuda* and therefore, that is so. This is how one can demonstrate the fault of *satpratipakṣa*.

TEXT 126

वस्तुतस्तु साधुत्वाज्ञानं न हेतुः अवयवादिव्युत्पन्नेन भ्रमाद्यजन्यं पूर्वप्रयोगमज्ञात्वापि नवकाव्यादिप्रयोगात् ।

Translation

As a matter of fact, the knowledge of correctness is not the proper ground because one who knows the etymological sense, even without knowing the earlier usage, which is not produced by illusion etc. uses words in the case of new literary compositions.

TEXT 127

कुतस्तर्हि ग्रामगामादो नान्वयबोधः, असाधुत्वनिश्चयादिति ब्रूमः ।

Translation

Then, how is it that in the case of the word *grāmagāma* etc. there is no verbal understanding?

(Reply): We would say that, because of the confirmation of not being the state of correct.

TEXT 128

साधोरप्यसाधुत्वनिश्चयेनाबोधकत्वात् अभिनवकाव्यादौ नासाधुत्वनिश्चयः ।

Translation

And also because of the confirmation of the state of not being correct or word does not produce understanding.

In the case of the new literary compositions, however, there arises no confirmation of the state of not being correct.

TEXT 129

संशयश्च न प्रतिबन्धकः, अन्यथा योगरूढिसंशये सत्यभिनवव्यक्तौ पाचकादि-प्रयोगो न स्यात् ।

Translation

The doubt which arises is not the obstruction. Otherwise when doubt arises of a etymologico-conventional sense, there does not arise the usage of *pācaka* etc. with reference to a new individual (meaning).

TEXT 130

अन्ये तु ततोऽन्वयबोधो भवत्येव, अपभ्रंशादिव यथा तव साधुत्वभ्रमात्, साधुत्वं तस्य नास्ति तद्वदेव ।

Translation

Some are of the opinion that from that word there does arise the verbal understanding as from the *apabhraṁśa* words you have understanding on the basis of the illusion of correctness since there is no correctness in it.

TEXT 131

अपरे त्वत्राकांक्षैव नास्ति घटः कर्मत्वमानयनमित्यत्रैव ।

Translation

Others are of the opinion that, there is no expectancy when the words as in the case of *ghuṭaḥ* 'pot', *karmatva* 'the objectness' and *ānayana* 'the action of bringing' etc. (in place of *ghataṁ ānaya* 'bring the pot').

TEXT 132

यत्तु गमाद्यनुत्तराण्त्वेन गमादिपूर्वेतराण्त्वेन वा शक्तिः काशपूर्वेत्तर-कुशत्वेनेवेति ।

Translation

Indeed, in the case that, there is *śakti* in the suffix *aṇ*—which is not followed by the root *gam*—or in the *aṇ*—other than that which is earlier of the root *gam*—as it is in the form of (*kuśa-kāśa*) being *kuśa* other than that which is earlier of the *kāśa*.

TEXT 133

तन्न। कर्मोपपद्धातुत्तराण्त्वेनैव शक्तेर्न तु तत्तद्धात्वनुत्तराण्त्वेन गौरवात् तत्तद्धातूनांविशिष्यज्ञाने शक्तिग्रहानुपपत्तेः कर्मण्यणिति सूत्रार्थमजानतः कुम्भकारादिपदप्रयोगानुपपत्तेश्च शक्तिसन्देहात्।

Translation

(Reply) : That is not tenable, because the *śakti* in *aṇ*—which is not followed by the root and which is adjacent to a form ending in accusative but not in *aṇ*—which is not followed from that root, which is cumbersome.

And also because in the absence of the knowledge of specific roots, there does not arise the knowledge of *śakti* and hence without knowing the meaning of the *sūtra*-'*karmaṇi aṇ*-' there will not arise the usage of the compound word' *kumbhakāra* because there is doubt in accepting *śakti*.

TEXT 134

असाधुत्वंच न भ्रमादिजन्यत्वं अनाप्तोक्ते असाधुत्वापत्तेः शुकाद्युदीरिते ग्रामगामादौ भ्रमाद्यजन्यत्वाच्च। किन्तु महाजनपरिगृहीतव्याकरणस्मृतिनिषिद्धत्वं तदपरिगृहीतत्वं वेति वक्ष्यते।

Translation

The state of not being correct is not the state of being produced by illusion, because when it is not uttered by the believable person, there will arise the contingency of not being correct and also because the word *grāmagāma* being uttered by a parrot, there is the state of not being produced by illusion.

But (*asādhutva*, means) the state of not being correct as per the norms of grammatical rule which is accepted by the well-formed persons, or (*asādhutva* means) the state of not being accepted by the elite. This we shall discuss in course of time.

TEXT 135

पदस्य साधुत्वं वृत्तिरेव। वत्तिश्च शाब्दबोधहेतुपदार्थोपस्थितत्तनुकुलपद-पदार्थयो: सम्बन्ध:।

Translation

The correctness of a word is the *vṛtti* and the *vṛtti* also means the relation between the word and its meaning which causes the presenting of the meaning and which is the cause of verbal understanding.

TEXT 136

वाक्यसाधुत्वंचाकांक्षादिमत्स्वार्थान्वयबोधकत्वे सति व्याकरणस्मृत्य-निषिद्धत्वम्।

Translation

And the correctness of a sentence means possessing expectancy etc., which is expressive of the relation with its own word-meaning and not being prohibited by the grammatical rules.

TEXT 137

तस्मात् कुमुदे पंकजशब्दस्य साधुत्वे सति प्रयोगप्रतिबन्धकत्वेन समुदाय-शक्तिसिद्धिरिति।

Translation

Therefore, although the word *paṅkaja* is correct it is not used in the sense of *kumuda*, and hence the *samudāyaśakti* is established.

TEXT 138

न चैवं लाघवात् जशब्द एव शक्तिरस्तु न समुदाये, मन्दुरजादौ पद्मधी-प्रसङ्गात्।

Translation

One cannot argue that, due to logical simplicity, let the word *ja*—only be treated as having *śakti*, but not in the whole word, because there will arise the contingency of the knowledge of lotus in the case of the word *Manduraja* 'one who is born in a stable'.

TEXT 139

पंकोत्तरजपदत्वेन शक्तिरिति चेत्तर्हि सर्वत्र तत्तद्वर्णोत्तरान्त्यवर्ण एव शक्ति-रिति समुदायशक्त्युच्छेदः ।

Translation

If somebody argues that the *śakti* will be accepted in the word *ja*—when it comes after the word *paṅka*, then in all cases there will be *śakti* in last letters which come after those every letters and there will be no necessity of accepting *samudāya-śakti* at all.

TEXT 140

न चैवं, विनिगमकाभावादिति सम्प्रदायः ।

Translation

It is also not the case, that since there is no proper alternative and so that position should be accepted. This is the traditional stand.

TEXT 141

अत्र ब्रूमः ज्ञाता हि या शक्यमनुभावयति सा शक्तिः ।

Translation

Here is our answer, that which is being known expresses the meaning (through some relation) is called *śakti*.

TEXT 142

न च समुदायः पद्मानुभवहेतुः, अवयवादेव तदुपपत्तेः ।

Translation

One cannot argue that, *samudāyaśakti* is the cause of the experience of lotus, because through *avayavaśakti*, that experience alone is possible.

TEXT 143

एवंच प्रतिबन्धकमात्रे शक्तिपदं पारिभाषिकम् ।

Translation

Thus, the word *śakti* is technical with reference to obstructor in general.

TEXT 144

शक्तित्वादनुभावकत्वसाधनेऽन्योन्याश्रयः प्रतिबन्धकत्वेनावगते शक्तित्वासिद्धिश्च ।

Translation

But if *śakti* is established as the causer of the understanding there will be mutual dependency, and if it is understood as an obstructor, *śakti* is not established.

TEXT 145

मण्डपादौ त्वनुभावकत्वेनैवशक्तिसिद्धिः ।

Translation

In the case of the word *maṇḍapa* etc., *śakti* is established as being the causer of experience.

TEXT 146

किञ्च रूढियोगयोर्विरोध एव परं रूढ्या योगप्रतिबन्धः मण्डपादौ तथा निर्णयात् । अन्यथा लम्बकर्णादावपि योगप्रतिवन्धः स्यात् ।

Translation

Moreover, there is contradiction between *rūḍhi* and *yoga* and then through conventional meaning the etymological meaning is obstructed, that we have already decided in connection with the word *maṇḍapa* earlier.

Otherwise, in the case of the word *lambakarṇa* there should be no obstruction of etymological sense.

TEXT 147

न चेह विरोधः, पद्मे समावेशात् योगादर्थधीश्चोभयत्र तुल्या ।

Translation

There is no difficulty here, because by the inclusion in lotus

TEXT 18

on the basis of etymology the knowledge of its meaning is possible and hence both are on par.

TEXT 148

यत्तु पंकजमानयेत्यादौ रूढ्या शीघ्रोपस्थितं पद्ममेव क्रिययान्वीयते, न पद्मजन्मकर्तृ, तस्य वाक्यार्थत्वेन विलम्बितप्रतीतीकत्वात् ।

Translation

Indeed, in the case of the sentence—*paṅkajam ānaya* 'bring the lotus', through conventional sense, the meaning 'lotus' is immediately remembered and is related with the action of bringing but not 'that what grows in the mud' because that is the sentence meaning and hence delayed.

TEXT 149

एवञ्चाविरोधेऽपि रूढिर्योगापहारितेति ।

Translation

And thus, if it is said that, since there is no contradiction, that the conventional meaning dominates over the etymological meaning.

TEXT 150

तन्न । क्रियापदतदर्थयोग्यतादिज्ञानाधीनत्वेन क्रियान्वयबोधस्य विलम्बितत्वात् । रूढ्यवयवार्थयोरन्वयबोधस्य सामग्रीसत्त्वेन प्राथमिकत्वात् । तस्मान्न प्रतिबन्धकत्वेन रूढिसिद्धिर्न वा तया योगप्रतिबन्ध इति ।

Translation

(Reply) : That is not tenable, because the verbal understanding is delayed, because it depends on the knowledge of root and its meaning by the help of the knowledge of the compatibility etc. and also because the understanding of both the meanings by *rūḍhi* and *yoga*, the factors being present immediately appears in the process of verbal understanding.

Therefore, the *rūḍhi* is established neither as an obstructor nor the *yoga* is obstructed by it.

TEXT 151

अत्रोच्यते। नियमतः पद्मस्मृत्यर्थमेव रूढिः, रूढ्या च नियमतः स्मृतं पद्ममेवावयवैः पंकजनिकर्तृत्वेनानुभाव्यते, बाधकं विनाव्यक्तिवचनानां सन्निहितविशेषपरत्वनियमात्।

Translation

Thus, it can be answered in the following manner : *rūḍhi* is for the regular remembrance of the meaning 'lotus' and through *rūḍhi*, regularly one experiences the remembered lotus only and through the etymology one experiences 'that which grows in the mud', because there is a rule that without an obstruction the words expressing the particular individuals stand for the particular meaning which is adjacent to it.

TEXT 152

अतः सर्वत्र पद्मानुभवसामग्र्येवेति न कुमुदे धीप्रयोगौ।

Translation

That is why in all cases (of the usage of the word *paṅkaja*), there arises the experience of 'lotus' through auxiliary factors, but the knowledge and the usage do not arise with reference to 'lily'.

TEXT 153

न चैवमनुभवाजनकत्वेन न सा शक्तिः या ज्ञाता नियमतः शक्यं ज्ञापयति सैव हि शक्तिः ज्ञप्तिश्च स्मृतिरनुभूतिश्चेति नियतस्मारिकापि शक्तिः।

Translation

It cannot be said that is not *śakti* and that what is known and regularly expresses its meaning alone is *śakti*, and the knowledge is of two types—remembrance and experience. Therefore, that which regularly reminds the meaning is also called *śakti*.

TEXT 154

वस्तुतः स्वार्थस्मृतिद्वारा अबयवानामिव समुदायस्य स्वार्थानुभावकत्वमविशेषादिति, पश्चादनुभाविकापि रूढिः, पंकजमानयेत्यादावानयनादिना स्वार्थान्वयानुभवे समुदायावयवयोर्हेतुत्वाच्च। तस्मान्नियतस्मृतिहेतुत्वेनैव रूढिसिद्धिः न तु प्रतिबन्धकत्वेन।

Translation

Really speaking, by the remembrance of one's own meaning like the *avayavaśakti* the *samudāyaśakti* also is the causer of the experience of its own meaning as there is no specific ground.

And then *rūḍhi* is also treated as the experiencer, because in the case of the sentence, *paṅkajam ānaya*, by the action of bringing in the experience of its own meaning since *samudāyaśakti* as well as *avayavaśakti* both being causes.

Therefore, on the basis of the ground of the regular remembrance of the meaning *rūḍhi* is established but not as an obstructor (of the primary sense).

TEXT 155

यदि च नियता स्मृतिः प्रकान्तरेण भवति तदा योग एव न रूढिः। रूढिन्यायेनैव कुमुदे धीप्रयोगयोरभावादिति। गोपदस्य गवि वेदेऽहीनपदस्य कर्मविशेषे रूढिरेव लाघवात्।

Translation

And if also the regular remembrance is possible through other means then it is a case of *yoga* but not *rūḍhi*.

Because, by the rule *yogād rūḍhir balīyasī*, with reference to *kumuda*, there is no knowledge and usage; the word *go* stands for 'cow' and in the *Veda* the word *ahīna* is used in the sense of a sacrifice, because it is logically simpler.

Notes

Rūḍhinyāya: The *nyāya* runs as follows : *yogād rūḍhir balīyasī*, *rūḍhi* i.e. the conventional relation is stronger than the *yoga* i.e. the etymological relation.

When a word has both possibilities of understanding arising either through *avayavaśakti* or through *samudāyaśakti*, in such case the *samudāyaśakti* works quickly and the meaning is remembered but not the etymological sense through *avayavaśakti*.

For example, the word *kuśala* etymologically means *kuśān lāti iti* 'one who collects *kuśa* grass 'but conventionally the word is used for a skilled person. When both possibilities are there, one is reminded of the conventional meaning first and understands as 'a skilled person' but not the etymological sense of it. It is because the *samudāyaśakti* i.e. *rūḍhi* predominates over the *avayavaśakti* i.e. *yoga.*

TEXT 156

न तु गमेर्डोंरन्हः खः क्रतावित्यनुशासनाद्योगेऽपि, डोः खप्रत्यययोर्लोके कर्त्तरि कर्मविशेषे च शक्तिर्न क्लृप्ता अतः प्रत्यये शक्तिनियामकञ्च गमिपदोत्तरत्वमहः पदोत्तरत्वञ्च कल्प्यं, तथाच गौरवम् ।

Translation

It is not proper to argue that from the *uṇādi sūtras gamer ḍoḥ, ahnaḥ khaḥ. kratau dābhābhyām nuḥ* etc. there is etymology also because in ordinary usage the suffixes *ḍa, kha* etc. are not used to convey an agent and a particular sacrifice and hence *śakti* is not established here in the suffixes.

One should postulate the regulating factor in the suffixes namely, 'being subsequent to the root *gam-*' and being subsequent to the word *ahar*, and this will lead to cumbersomeness.

TEXT 157

एवं धैनुपदेऽप्येकैकस्यातिप्रसक्तत्वात् गोत्वविशिष्टधानकर्मणि रूढिरेव नियमतो गोत्वविशिष्टोपस्थितेः, न तु योगोऽपि, दानु-भानु कृशान्वादौ भिन्नार्थत्वेन नुप्रत्ययशक्तेरकल्पनान् गमेर्डोरन्हः खः क्रतौ दा-भाभ्यां नुर्धेटइच्चेत्यादिस्मृतिश्चालवड्डादिवत् कथञ्चिद्व्युत्पादनपरा ।

Translation

Likewise, in the word *dhenu* also, since there is logical inconsistency expresses through *rūḍhi* 'that which is an object of milking and which possesses cowness', because regularly one is reminded of that which possesses *gotva*, but not through *yoga* also.

In the case of the words like *dānu*, *bhānu* and *kṛuśānu* etc., since there is difference in meanings, one cannot postulate *śakti* in the suffix *nu*—but by the knowledge of the grammatical rules *gamer ḍoḥ, ahnaḥ khaḥ kratau dābhābhyām nuḥ, dheṭa it ca* etc., like the word *alavaḍḍa* etc., somehow one finds the etymology.

Notes

Alavaḍḍa : Mathurānātha Tarkavâgiśa in his *Ālokarahasya* says that—*kāṣṭha pratimākāra vācitvam*, that means—'which is expressive of a statue made of wood'. But Pakṣadhara Mishra in his *āloka* says that one finds the etymology somehow like—*alavat taṁ ḍāti kṣipatiti*. Mathurānātha, however, does not favour the etymological meaning.

TEXT 158

अतएव भगवान् पाणिनिरर्थाननुगमात् समुदायशक्त्यपेक्षया गौरवादुणादिप्रत्ययेषु न शक्तिरिति, पञ्चपादिकाविहितानुणादिप्रत्ययान् उणादयो बहुलमित्येकेनैव सूत्रेण विहितवान्, यत्र तु प्रत्यये शक्तिस्तत्र प्रत्येकमेवासूत्रयत् ।

Translation

Therefore, the great teacher *Pāṇini*, since the different meanings cannot be brought under one group in comparison to the *samudāyaśakti* enjoined the suffixes which are not enjoined in the *pañcapādikā*, by the rule *uṇādayo vahulam* since there is no *śakti* in *uṇādi* suffixes, where there is *śakti* in the suffix, there he composed each *sūtra* separately.

TEXT 159

यत्तु धेनुपदे गोत्वं न शक्यं, किन्तु शक्योपलक्षणतया शक्त्युपाधिः, यत्र गोत्वं तद्धानकर्म शक्यं शक्यास्तूपलक्ष्या महिष्यादिव्यावृत्ता धानकर्मव्यक्तिविशेषाएव, अनुगमस्तूपलक्षणैक्यात् ।

Translation

There was the following view : cowness is not the expressed sense of the word *dhenu*, but merely an *upādhi* being an indicator of the expressed sense.

Where there is cowness, that is the object of milking and that expressed senses are implied and are excluded from buffaloes etc. and are the particular objects of milking and they are brought into one group because there is unity in indication.

TEXT 160

न चैवं लाघवाद्गोत्वं शक्यं धानकर्मत्वमुपाधिः, उपलक्ष्यस्य गोत्वस्याति-

प्रसक्तत्वात् । गोत्वविशिष्टधानस्मृतिस्त्वेकैव शब्दसंस्काराभ्यां जन्यते न तूभय-स्मृत्यनन्तरं परस्परमन्वयबोधः अवयवशक्तेरभावादिति ।

Translation

It is not proper to argue that, due to logical simplicity let cowness be the expressed sense and the object of milking be an *upādhi* because that cowness which is indicated will lead to the state of over-application which is logically inconsistent.

And also because the remembrance of milking which is qualified by cowness is one and is produced by both a word (cow) and the impression, but not after the remembrance of both, there arises the verbal understanding of the mutual relationship because there is no *avayavaśakti.*

TEXT 161

तन्न । शक्तिं विना नियतगोत्वोपस्थित्यभावादुपलक्षणैक्येन उपलक्ष्यैक्या-भावाच्च । अन्यथा महिष्यादिव्यावृत्तधानकर्मत्वेऽपि न शक्तिः धान-गोत्वे शक्त्युपाधी, अग्रे च संस्कारादुपस्थितयोस्तयोः कर्मणि धेनुपदादन्वयोभासत इति धानमपि न शक्यम् । यदि चानुततं विशेषणं शक्त्युपाधिर्विशेष्ये च शक्तिरननुगमा-तिप्रसंगाभावश्चोपाधिनैव, तदौपाधिककारणादिपदानां विशिष्टे शक्तिर्न स्यात् ।

Translation

(*Reply*) : It is not tenable because without *śakti* there does not arise the regular remembrance of cowness and it is not true that through the unity of indication there is unity of indicated. Otherwise, there is no *śakti* in the object of milking excluded from buffalo etc. and both the object of milking and cowness should be the *upādhi* of the *śakti.* And since the understanding arises of the relation of both the object of milking and cowness remembered through impression, the object of milking is also not to be treated as the expressed sense.

If it is said that the consecutive qualifier is the *upādhi* of *śakti* and there is *śakti* with reference to the qualificand and by *upādhi* itself the meanings could be brought into one group and there will not be any contingency of over-application, then there should not be *śakti* with reference to the qualified in case of the words like *aupādhika-kāraṇa* etc.

TEXT 162

नन्ववयवात् पंकजनिकर्तृत्वानुभवः समुदायाच्च पद्मस्मरणं स्यात् । न तु पंकजनिकर्तृ पद्ममित्यनुभव इति चेत् ।

Translation

Well, if it is argued that, through *avayavaśakti* there arises the experience of 'that which grows in the mud' and through *samudāyaśakti*, there will arise the remembrance of lotus (from the word *paṅkaja*), but not the experience of 'lotus which grows in the mud'.

TEXT 163

न, अवयव-समुदायस्मारितपंकजनिकर्तृ पद्मानां पंकजनिकर्तृ पद्ममित्यनुभवोऽवयव-समुदायाभ्यां सम्भूय जन्यते, समुदायोपस्थितपद्मेन समं स्वार्थान्वयोऽवयवैर्वा अवयवजनितानुभवोपस्थितपंकजनिर्तृत्वेन समं स्वार्थान्वयः वा अनुभाव्यते, आकांक्षाद्युपेतशब्दानां तात्पर्यविषयोपस्थापितस्वार्थान्वयबोधकत्वनियमात् ।

Translation

(Reply) : It is not acceptable, because the knowledge of lotus which grows in the mud is produced by both *avayavaśakti* and *samudāyaśakti* together, as lotus which grows in the mud being remembered by *avayava śakti* and *samudāyaśakti*.

And also because, the relationship with its meaning is known either by *avayavaśakti* with reference to the lotus which is presented by *samudāyaśakti*, or, the relationship with its meaning is experienced through *samudāyaśakti* with reference to the experience which is presented by that which grows in the mud, which is produced by the *avayavaśakti*, because there is a rule that the words having expectancy etc. cause the knowledge of the relationship with their meanings presented by the intention of the speaker.

TEXT 164

न च वाक्यान्तरे तथात्वादर्शनेन नैवं व्युत्पत्तिरिति वाच्यम ।

Translation

It cannot be argued that, in other sentences as the knowledge of relationship is not seen there is no etymology of that type possible.

TEXT 165

वाक्यान्तरे हि समुदायशक्त्यभावेन तथा, अत्र तु समुदायशक्तिवलात् पदविधया वाक्यविधया वा एकस्मादेवोपस्थितयोः पंकजनिकर्तृ-पद्मयोरन्वयो बोध्यते समुदायेन पदैकवाक्यतावत् पंकज कुमुदमित्यत्र समुदायेनैवपंकजनिकर्तृत्वमशक्यं स्वार्थपद्मसम्बन्धि लक्ष्यते। कुमुदे साधुत्वात् कथं तत्र लक्षणेति चेत्, न, समुदायस्य तत्रासाधुत्वात्।

Translation

Because in other sentences as there is no *samudāyaśakti* but in the present case, on the strength of *samudāyaśakti* either in the form of a word or a sentence the relationship is known from one expression when presented in both forms like that which grows in the mud and lotus like the sentence unity through *samudāyaśakti*. In the sentence *paṅkajam kumudam* (*ānaya*) through *samudāyaṣakti* only 'that which grows in the mud' is not an expressed sense and is indicated by its own meaning which is related to lotus.

If it is argued that in *kumuda*, since there is correctness how is there *lakṣaṇā* in that word?

It is not true because there is *asādhutva* with reference to the *samudāyaśakti*.

Notes

Vākyaikavākyatā :

This concept is used in the Mīmāṁsā system. When the expressed meanings of two different sentences are fit to be united to each other with reference to their meanings and being related they form one sentence and convey one sense. That is called *vākyaikavākyatā*. For example : there are two injunctions—"*Agnihotram juhuyāt svargakāmaḥ* and *Dadhnā juhoti.*"

Now both these sentences have separate meanings independently and prescribe some action to be performed. Still they have an expectancy of each other. The first sentence prescribes the sacrifice to be performed but nothing is mentioned about the process, how and with what he should perform the sacrifice.

On the other hand the second sentence prescribes that one has to offer curds in the sacrifice but he does not know with reference to what sacrifice he has to offer curds and for what purpose.

In such case, if both sentences are read together as a single sentence they will express a complete meaning—this type of sentence unity is called *vākyaikavākyatā.*[1]

Padikavākyatā :

This concept also comes under the sentence unity (*ekavākyatā*) in Mīmāṁsā system. The problem starts with how the *arthavāda* sentences are to be connected with *vidhi* sentences. And hence it is solved by the process of *padaikavākyatā.*

There are some *arthavāda* sentences namely: *vāyur vai kṣepiṣṭhā devatā, vāyum eva svena bhāgadheyena abhidhāvati, sa eva enam bhūtim gamayati.*

And there is another sentence which prescribes a sacrifice namely—'*vāyavyam śvetam ālabheta bhūtikāmaḥ*'.

The first set of sentences refer to a praise of the deity *vāyu* but do not express any action to be performed. It is natural that this praise has an expectancy towards some sentence which expresses some action which has *Vāyu* as its deity.

On the other hand, the second sentence has an expectancy of some praise that will instigate the person to undertake the action enjoined by it.

If both expressions are connected, then they will express a complete meaning and induce a person to take up the sacrifice. But how to connect these two expressions namely—the *vidhi* and the *arthavāda* ?

---

1. *Panse*, Ujjvala, *A Reconstruction of the Third School of Pūrvamīmāṁsā*, p. 76.

So by *lakṣaṇā* the *arthavāda* sentence will expresses *prāsastya* i.e. praise of the sacrifice which is just a word meaning. In this way the *arthavāda* sentence is brought to the level of a word and then the *prāśastya* gets connected with the *vidhi* sentence. Thus, the united sentence expresses the praised sacrifice that is to be performed. This type of sentence unity is called as *padaikavākyatā*[1] i.e. unity of a sentence with a *pada*.

TEXT 166

यत्तु तत्र पद्मत्वमयोग्यतया नान्वेति योगादेव मुख्यया वृत्त्या कुमुदे पंकजनिकर्तृत्वमनुभूयते इति तन्न, कुमुदेऽवयवशक्तेः समुदायशक्त्या ज्ञातया प्रतिबन्धात् तथैव तदवगमात् ।

Translation

There was a view that since lotusness is not compatible it is not related to *kumuda* on the basis of *yoga* i.e. the primary relationship, there arises the knowledge of that which grows in the mud from the word *kumuda*.

(*Reply*) : It is not tenable because the *avayavaśakti* in the word *kumuda* is obstructed by the *samudāyaśakti* which is known and also because that word *kumuda* is known like that.

TEXT 167

ननु यदा व्यक्तिवचनन्यायात् न कुमुदे धीर्नं त्ववयवशक्तिप्रतिबन्धात् तदा पंकजशब्दादुपस्थिते पंकजं पद्ममिति वाक्यार्थेऽयोयतया पद्ममपहाय पदवाक्यैकवाक्यतया पंकजनिकर्तृ कुमुदमित्यनुभव इति चेत् ।

Translation

Well, when by the rule that the word expresses a particular individual, there does not arise the knowledge with reference to *kumuda*, because the *avayavaśakti* obstructs it, in such case then the knowledge that arises is that *paṅkajam padmam* from the word *paṅkaja* and since it is not compatible with the sentence meaning by removing *padma* by the sentence unity of a word

Ibid.

and sentence if it is said that, there arises the knowledge of *kumuda* which grows in the mud.

TEXT 168

तर्हिपद्मान्वितत्वेनोपस्थितस्य पंकजनिकर्तृत्वस्याश्रयाकांक्षा नास्तीति स्वतन्त्रोपस्थित्यर्थंमवश्यं लक्षणा, यथा पुरोडाशकपालपदेऽधिष्ठानलक्षणा ।

Translation

Then there is no need of taking resort to expectancy of that which grows in the mud which is presented by the relationship with reference to lotus and hence one should accept *lakṣaṇā* for understanding separately (for the word *kumuda*) as in the case of the word *puroḍāśakapāla*, the deity is known through *lakṣaṇā* only.

TEXT 169

ननु प्रथममेवावयव-कुमुदपदै रन्वययोग्यतया स्मृतं पद्मं त्यक्त्वास्वार्थान्वया-नुभव इति चेत् ।

Translation

Well, if it is argued that, through the *avayavaśakti, kumuda* is compatible with its relationship and having kept aside the remembered meaning lotus, there is the knowledge of its relationship with its own meaning.

TEXT 170

कुमुदपद-तदर्थयोग्यतादिज्ञानात् पूर्वमेव पंकजशब्दात् पंकजं पद्ममित्यनु-भवात् विलम्बे हेत्वभावात्, स्थलपंकजन्तु विजातीयमेव, साजात्येऽपि तत्र लक्षणा ।

Translation

(*Reply*) : (It is not true), Because before the knowledge of the compatibility with its own meaning of the word *kumuda* since there is the earlier knowledge that *paṅkaja* is *padma* from the word *paṅkaja* there is no ground of being delayed.

But in the case of the word *sthalapadma*, it is treated as of different class, while belonging to same class (like *kumuda*), there is *lakṣaṇā*.

TEXT 171

यत्तु अयोग्यतया योगार्थोनान्वेति किन्तु योग्यतया रूढ्युपस्थितं पद्मत्व-मेवान्वीयते इति ।

Translation

Indeed, since there is incompatibility the etymological sense is not known but by compatibility lotusness is conveyed which is presented by *rūḍhi*.

TEXT 172

तन्न । पद्मत्वस्य यौगार्थगतत्वेन उपस्थित्या निराकांक्षत्वात् । स्वतन्त्रोप-स्थितये लक्षणया अवश्यं वाच्यत्वादिति ।

Translation

(*Reply*) : It is also not tenable, because lotusness is known by the etymological sense and by its presence it is not desired. The secondary relation ts necessary in order to have independent remembrance of meaning.

Bibliography

I. Primary Sources
II. Secondary Sources

I. PRIMARY SOURCES

Kārikāvalī—Muktāvalī of Viśvanātha Nyāyapañcānana with *Dīnakarī* and *Rāmarudrī*. Ed. by Sri Harirama Sukla, Chaukhamba Sanskrit Series Gupta Office, Varanasi, 1951.

Kavyālaṁkāra sūtra vṛttiḥ, Oriental Book Agency, Poona, 1927.

Kiraṇāvalī, Ed. by Gourinath Shastri, Sampurnanda Sanskrit Vishvavidyalaya, Varanasi, 1980.

Tattvacintāmaṇi (*Śabdakhaṇḍa*), with Comm. *Āloka* and *Rahasya*, Ed. by Pt. Kāmākhyānāth Tankavāgīśa, Bibliotheca Indica, Asiatic Society, 1897.

Tattvārtha Sūtra of Umāsvāti, Ed. by Mohanlal Mehta, Parsvanath Vidyashrama Research Institute, Varanasi, 1985.

Tarka Kaumudī of Laugākṣibhāskara, Ed. by K.N. Chatterjee, Chowkhamba Amarabharati Prakashan, Varanasi, 1982.

Tarkabhāṣā of Keśava Miśra, Ed. by S.R. Iyer, Chaukhambha Orientalia, Varanasi, 1979.

Tarkasaṁgraha of Annambhaṭṭa with *Tarkadīpikā* and Govardhana's *Nyāyabodhinī*, Ed. by Y.V. Athalye and M.R. Bodas, Bombay Sanskrit Series No. LV, Bhandarkar Oriental Research Institute, Poona-4, 1930.

Tarkāmṛta with *vivṛti* commentary, The Asiatic Society. Calcutta, 1974.

Nirukta, Ed. by Lakshman Sarup, Motilal Banarsidass, 1967.

Nītitattvāvirbhāva, Ed. by P.K. Narayana Pillai, University of Travancore, Trivandrum Sanskrit Series, No. 168, Trivandrum, 1953.

Nīlakaṇṭhī, by Nīlakaṇṭhabhaṭṭa, Published from Banaras, 187[illegible].

Nyāyakośa, Ed, by M.M. Bhimācārya Jhalakikar, Revised and re-edited by Vāsudev Shastri Abhyankar, Bombay Sanskrit Series, Bhandarkar Oriental Research Institute, Poona, 1978.

Nyāyadarśanam with *Bhāṣya*, *vārttika*, *tātparyaṭīkā*, and *vṛtti*, Ed. by Tārānāth Nyāya Tarkatīrtha and Amarendramohan Tarkatīrtha, Munshiram Manoharlal Publishers Pvt. Ltd., 2nd edition, 1985.

Nyāyapradīpa by Gangasahāya Sharma, Shree Venketeswar Press, Bombay, 1907.

Nyāyabinduprakaraṇam with *Tīkā*, Ed. by, Swami Dwarika Das Shastri, Bauddha Bharati, Varanasi, 1985.

Nyāyabhūṣaṇam, Ed. by Swami Yogindrananda, Śaḍdars'an Prakashan Pratisthanam, Varanasi, 1968.

Nyāyamañjarī (Part I & II) with *ṭippaṇinyāyasaurabha*, Ed. by K.S. Varadacharya, Oriental Research Institute, Mysore, 1969.

Nyāyamālāvistāra on *Jaiminīyanyāyamālā* of Mādhavācārya, Ed. by Shivadatta Sharma, Anandashram Sanskrit Series, No. 24, poona, 1946.

Nyāyasiddhāntadīpa of Śaśadhara with *Tīppaṇa* by Guṇaratna Suri, Ed. by Bimal Krishna Matilal, L.D. Institute of Indology, Ahmedabad, 1976.

Nyāyasiddhānta-dīpa Prabhā a comm. on *Nyāya Siddhānta Dīpa* by Śeśānanta, *The Pandit*, Vol. XLI, Benaras, 1919.

Paramalaghumañjūṣā with the commentary *Jyotsnā*, Ed. by Kālikāprasād Śukla, Baroda Sanskrit Mahavidyalaya, Baroda, 1961.

Pātañjala Yogadarśana containing *yogasūtra*, *yogabhāṣya*, *Tattvavisāradī* and *yogavārttika*, Varanasi, 1971.

Prakaraṇapañcikā with *Nyāya-siddhi*, Ed. by Mīmāṁsaratnam Pt. A. Subrahmanya Sastri, Banaras Hindu University, Banaras. 1961.

Praśastapādabhāṣya with *Nyāyakandalī*, Ed. by Durgadhara Jha, Sampurnanda Sanskrit Vishvavidyalaya, Varanasi, 1977.

Baudha Tarkabhāṣā, Ed. by Raghunath Giri, Prachyaprakashan, Varanasi—2, 1969.

Brahmasūtra Śankara Bhāṣya with *Bhāmatī*, *Kalpataru* and *Parimala*, Ed. by K.L. Joshi, Parimal Publications, Delhi, 1981.

Bhāṭṭacintāmaṇi on *Mīmāṁsā sūtra* by Visvesvara (Gāgā) Bhaṭṭa, with the Commentary *Mayūkha*, Ed. by Suryanarayana Shukla, Chaukhamba Sanskrit Series, Work No. 6,490, 1933, 1938.

Bhāṭṭadīpikā on *Mīmāṁsāsūtra* of Khaṇḍadeva, Ed. by A. Mahadeva Shastri and L. Srinivasacharya, Bibliotheca Sanskrita, Govt. Oriented Library Publications, Mysore, BS, 1908-1916.

Mahābhāṣya, Ed. by F. Keilhorn, Third Edn, Revised and furnished with additional readings, references and select critical notes by MM. K.V. Abhyankar, Vol. I, II and III, Bhandarkar Oriental Research Institute, Poona, 1962-72.

Mānameyodaya of Nārāyaṇa, Ed. by C. Kunhan Raja and S.S. Suryanarayana Shastri, Adyar, 1933.

Mīmāṁsākoṣa, Ed. by Kevelānanda Saraswatī, Prājñapāṭhaśālā Maṇḍalagranthamālā, Wai, 1952-66.

Mīmāṁsādarśana, Ed. by K.V. Abhyankar and G.S. Joshi, with *Tantravārttika*, Anandashram Sanskrit Series, No. 17, 1953-74.

Mīmāṁsāślokavārttika with Commentary *Kāśikā* (Part III), Ed. by V.A. Ramaswami Sastri, Trivandrum Sanskrit Series No. CL, University of Trivandrum, 1943.

Rasagaṅgādhara with Commentary of *Nāgeśa* and *Saralā of* Mathurānāth Sastri, Kāvyamālā, 12, 1947.

Laghuśabdendu Śekhara of Nāgeśa Bhaṭṭa, Vol. I, with the commentary *Śekharadīpaka* of Nityānanda Panta Parvatiya, Ed. by—Gopal Śastri Nene, Vol. II, Ed. by Narahari Sastri Pendse, KSS. 27, 1954, KSS. 5, 1922.

Vākyapadīya, Ed. by K.V. Abhyankar and V.P. Limaye, University of Poona Sanskrit and Prakrit Series, Vol. II, Poona, 1965.

Vaiyākarṇabhūṣaṇasāra with *Kāśikā* of Harirāma Kāla, Ed. by Kamalāsankara Prāṇaśankara Trivedi, Bombay Sanskrit and Prakrit Series—70, 1915.

Vaiyākaraṇa Siddhānta Laghumañjūṣā with the Commentary *Ratnaprabhā*, Ed. by Sabhāpati Śarmā Upādhyāya, Chaukhamba Sanskrit Series Office, Varanasi, 1963.

Vaiśeṣikadarśana with *Vedabhāskarabhāṣyam.* by Kashinath Sharma, Mandī (H.P.), 1972.

Vaiśeṣikasūtropaskāra with commentary *Prakāśikā*, Ed. by Narayana Mishra, Chaukhamba Sanskrit Series Office, Varanasi, 1969.

Vyutpattivāda with the commentary *Gūḍhārthatattvāloka* of Baccā Jha, Ed. by Hariraj, Harinath and Ramapati, Nirnaya Sagar Press, 1911.

Śaktivādaḥ of Gadādhara Bhaṭṭācārya with *Vivṛtti* of Harinatha Tarkasiddhanta Bhattacharya, Kashi, Sanskrit Series, No. 77, Chaukhamba Sanskrit Series Office, Varanasi, 1929.

Śabdaśaktiprakāśikā with two commentaries *Kṛṣṇakāntī* and *Probodhinī*, Ed. by Dhundiraj Shastri, Chaukhamba Sanskrit Series Office, Varanasi, 1973.

Śāstra Dīpikā Ed. by Kishoredas Swami, Sri Sadhubela Samskrit College, Benaras, 1977.

Ślokavārttika with Commentary *Nyāyaratnākara*, Ed. by Swami Dvārikādāsa Sāstri, Tara Publications, Varanasi, 1978.

Sarasvatīkaṇṭhābharaṇam with Commentary *Ratnadarpaṇam* Ed. by Kameshwaranath Mishra, Chaukhamba Orientalia, Varanasi, 1976.

Sarva-Darśana-Saṁgraha with a Commentary. Ed. by T.G. Mainkar, Bhandarkar Oriental Research Institute, Poona, 1978.

Sāṁkhyakārikā with *Anurādhā* Commentary of B.M. Chaturvedi, Delhi, 1969.

Sāṁkhyatattvakaumudī, Bombay, 1940.

Siddhāntacandrodaya, Commentary on *Tarkasaṁgraha* by Śrikṛṣṇadhūajaṭidīkṣit, Nirnaya Sagar Press, Bombay, 1957.

II. SECONDARY SOURCES

Bhattacharya Gopikamohan, *Navya-Nyāya, Some Logical Problems in Historical Perspective*, Bharatiya Vidya Prakashan, Delhi, 1978.

Bijalwan, G.D, *Indian Theory of Knowledge*, Heritage Publishers, New Delhi, 1977.

Chatterjee, K.N, *Word and Its Meaning a New Perspective*, Chaukhamba Orientalia, Varanasi, 1980.

Chatterjee, Satischandra, *The Nyāya Theory of Knowledge* (2nd Edn.), University of Calcutta, Calcutta, 1950.

Devasthali, G V, *Mīmāṁsā : The Vākyaśāstra of Ancient India*, (Vol. I), Booksellers Publishing Company, Bombay, 1959.

Francis X. D'sa, S.J, *Śabdaprāmāṇyam in Śabara and Kumārila*, Publications of the De Nobili Research Library, Vienna, 1980.

Guha, Dinesh Chandra, *Navya Nyāya System of Logic*, Motilal Banarsidass, Delhi, 1979.

Ingalalli, R. I, *Sabdapramāṇa : An Epistemological Analysis*, Sri Satguru Publications, Delhi, 1988.

Jha Ganganath, *The Prabhākara School of Pūrvamīmāṁsā* Motilal Banarsidass, Delhi, 1978.

Jha, Harimohan, *Trends oj Linguistic Analysis in Indian Philosophy*, Chaukhambha Orientalia, Varanasi, 1981.

Jha, V.N, *The Logic of the Intermediate Causal Link*, Sri Satguru Publications, Delhi 1986.

Jha, V.N, *Studies in Language, Logic and Epistemology*, Pratibha Prakashan, Delhi, 1986.

Jha, V.N, *Viṣayatāvāda* of Harirāma Tarkālaṁkāra, Centre of Advanced Study in Sanskrit, University of Poona, Poona, 1987.

Jha V.N, *The Philosophy of Injunctions*, Pratibha Prakashan, Delhi, 1987.

Jha, V.N, *The Philosophy of Relations*, Sri Satguru Publications, Delhi, 1990.

Joshi, S.D. (Ed.), *Vyākaraṇa Mahābhāṣya (Samarthāhnika)*, Centre of Advanced Study in Sanskrit, University of Poona, Poona, 1968.

Joshi, S.D. (Ed.), *Proceedings of the Winter Institute of Ancient Indian theories on Sentence-meaning*, Centre of Advanced Study in Sanskrit, University of Poona, Poona, 1980.

Matilal, Bimal Krishna, *Logic Language and Reality*, Motilal Banarsidass, Delhi, 1985.

Panse, Ujjvala, *A Reconstruction of the Third School of Pūrva Mīmāṁsā*, Sri Satguru Publications, New Delhi, 1990.

Raja, K. Kunjunni, *Indian Theories of Meaning*, The Adyar Library and Research Centre, Madras, 1963.

Rao, V.S, *The Philosophy of a Sentence and Its Parts*, Munsiram Monoharlal, New Delhi, 1969.

Shastri, Gaurinath, *The philosophy of word and meaning*, Sanskrit College Research Series No. 5, Calcutta, 1959.

Shivkumar, *Sāmkhya-yoga Epistemology*, Eastern Book Linkers, Delhi, 1984.

Singh, B.N, *Indian Logic*, Asha Prakashan, Varanasi, 1988.

Ullmann, Stephen, *Words and Their Use*, Frederick Muller Ltd., London, 1963.

Ullmann, Stephen, *The Principles of Semantics*, Basil Blackwell, Oxford, 1963.

Ullmann, Stephen, *Language and Style*, Basil Blackwell, Oxford, 1964.

Vyas, R.T. (Ed.), *Journal of the Oriental Institute*, (Vol. 37) Oriental Institute, Baroda, 1988.

Index

ERRATA

Page	Line	Misprint	Correct form
7	5	Buddha	Bauddha
8	24	*kāraṇā*	*karaṇa*
14	29	*śṛuti*	*śruti*
15	4	on	or
17	5	*na sā smṛtiḥ*	*iti*
26	8	*phalastara*	*phalastatra*
27	25	patteren	pattern
29	13, 14, 16	Devadaṭṭaḥ	Devadattaḥ
30	8	ward	word
30	13	words	word
30	23	defining	of defining
31	24	*Tat Tika*	*Tat Tīka*
32	16	*śabdāhdyāhāra*	*śabdādhyāhāra*
36	6	*sakti*	*śakti*
44	5	*sambandhī*	*sambandhi*
100	33	*yogarūṅhī*	*yogarūḍhi*
108	4, 6, 30	*pankaja*	*paṅkaja*
116	13	*doḥ*	*ḍoḥ*
116	33	*ahnah*	*ahnaḥ*

Page	*Line*	*Misprint*	*Correct form*
139	2	कृलप्तत्वात्	कृल्प्तत्वात्
139	16	स्मृत्मर्थं	स्मृत्यर्थं
139	17	पद्माधुभव	पद्ममानुभव
139	26	पद्मादाय	पद्ममादाय
140	26	नियेयोद्बोधे	नियतोद्बोधे
141	4	य	न
142	6	*śakit*	*śakti*
144	29	यतु	यत्तु
145	23	पद्मानयेत्यादौ	पद्ममानयेत्यादौ
146	2	शाब्दपद्ानुभवे	शाब्देपद्मानुभवे
151	7	कलपयति	कल्पयति
151	8	शब्दार्तत्वात्	शब्दार्थत्वात्
154	23	पद्स्मृति-	पद्मस्मृति-
159	27	यद्वोपङ्कजवेन	यद्वोपङ्कजत्वेंन
160	21	पद्मप्रमौगस्य	पद्मप्रयोगस्य